"Dr. Caroline Leaf is a brilliant and prolific communication pathologist and cognitive neuroscientist. With over thirty years in research and study, she delves into *Cleaning Up Your Mental Mess* with these five simple steps to help reduce our anxieties, stress, and toxic thinking. There is no better time to introduce these strategies than now. She brings a wealth of scientific information to the table while breaking it down into layperson's terms to help you live life to the fullest, free from the struggles and the pain that may have plagued you for years. This book will read like a manual to guide you through the vicissitudes of life to a better and healthier place."

Bishop T. D. Jakes, *New York Times* bestselling author

"In this wonderful new book, Dr. Caroline Leaf will change your healthspan forever by empowering you with a simple five-part plan, guided by three decades of clinical practice, that will make you more mindful of maintaining your mental and physical health. Start reading and let the transformation begin!"

Dr. Rudolph E. Tanzi, *New York Times* bestselling author of *The Healing Self* and professor of neurology, Harvard Medical School

"For years I've taught leaders to guard their thinking above all else in life, because *how* a leader thinks determines *what* a leader will accomplish. Healthy discipline of the mind is essential for success in life, and Dr. Caroline Leaf provides a five-step roadmap for developing truly helpful mental discipline. Her new book, *Cleaning Up Your Mental Mess*, is rooted in decades of research and shows how the journey to healthier thinking is shorter than you might think—and available to anyone willing to take it."

Dr. John C. Maxwell, leadership and personal growth expert

"One of the things I love about Caroline is her help in understanding the difference in our 'brains' and our 'minds.' In this book she takes us the next step in making both of them work better, leading us to feeling and performing better. Thanks, Caroline."

Dr. Henry Cloud, *New York Times* bestselling
author and clinical psychologist

"*Cleaning Up Your Mental Mess* is a powerful new book that can change your life. Learning how to manage your mind is a critical skill that should be taught in school, yet rarely is. This book can help decrease suffering and help your overall outlook and mood. I highly recommend it."

Daniel G. Amen, MD, founder of Amen Clinics
and author of *The End of Mental Illness*

"As someone who appreciates the human brain and its infinite capacity for growth and change, I was very excited to read Dr. Leaf's new book. In *Cleaning Up Your Mental Mess*, she teaches you how to make the most of your powerful mind and take back control over your thinking to live your best life and reach your full potential."

Jim Kwik, CEO of Kwik Learning, *New York Times*
bestselling author of *Limitless*, and host of the
Kwik Brain podcast; www.JimKwik.com

"*Cleaning Up Your Mental Mess* is an amazing new book that will teach you to change your mind, and your life, for the better. It offers easy to follow, scientifically based steps that will help you regain control of your thinking and mental health, empowering you to take back control and clean up that mental mess!"

Dr. Josh Axe, founder of Ancient Nutrition and DrAxe.com,
author of the bestselling books *Keto Diet* and *Collagen
Diet* and upcoming book *Ancient Remedies*,
and host of *The Dr. Axe Show*

"Our mental health is being threatened like never before. Unfortunately, the pharmaceutical fixes that represent the central tools of modern medicine fall far short when it comes to such pervasive issues as anxiety, depression, and other challenges to mood and mental wellness. But there is a north star. In *Cleaning Up Your Mental Mess*, Dr. Caroline Leaf leverages over thirty years of clinical experience to offer us empowering, effective, and time-tested guidance for unraveling toxic stress and regaining control of our mental state, paving the way for happiness, satisfaction, and contentment. From both preventive and treatment perspectives, this book delivers on its promise."

David Perlmutter, MD, author of the #1 *New York Times* bestsellers *Grain Brain* and *Brain Wash*

"Ours is a society plagued by a lack of reflection and an over-abundance of destructive, quick-fix answers. In her new book, Dr. Caroline Leaf offers an antidote to these caustic thought patterns. By focusing on five practical steps to brain change, Dr. Leaf provides a pragmatic approach to sustainable wellness."

Austin Perlmutter, MD, coauthor of *New York Times* bestseller *Brain Wash*

"In times like these, *Cleaning Up Your Mental Mess* is a true gift. With a rise of anxiety, depression, and intrusive thoughts, Dr. Caroline Leaf delivers a scientifically tested system to navigate today's uncertain world. This book gives you paradigm-shifting insight on the brain, how it works, and how you can become an empowered participant in creating new neural pathways. Dr. Leaf is a pioneer in neuroscience and mental health, and I recommend this for everyone interested in creating their own destiny."

Dr. Nicole LePera, The Holistic Psychologist; yourholisticpsychologist.com; @the.holistic.psychologist

"*Cleaning Up Your Mental Mess* is an incredible new book that will teach you how to take back control over your thinking. Using her decades of research and clinical experience, Dr. Leaf shows the reader how they can, no matter where they are in life, harness the power in their mind to change their mental health and their life."

Frank Lipman, MD, Integrative Medicine

"In *Cleaning Up Your Mental Mess*, Dr. Caroline Leaf masterfully weaves the latest brain science and practical tips to help you take back control of your health and life. Not only will this book help you clean up the mess in your mind but it will help you start living your best life—so that you can start being all that you want to be."

Jason Wachob, founder and co-CEO, mindbodygreen

"As important as time management may be, the art of mind management is a lost ability that very few study and even fewer are able to teach. Dr. Leaf is one of the few who is able to teach this lost art."

Patrick Bet-David, author of #1 *Wall Street Journal* bestseller *Your Next Five Moves*

"My friend and esteemed colleague Dr. Caroline Leaf's *Cleaning Up Your Mental Mess* is the paradigm-breaking resource that will redefine the way we look at and address mental health. So many of us are perpetually stressed and anxious, and it plays out negatively in all areas of our lives, including our relationships and physical health. By utilizing over thirty years of clinical experience, Dr. Leaf provides us with a comprehensive yet practical guide to finally managing the clutter in our minds with science-based tools that actually work. Here's to cleaning up all of our mental mess!"

Dr. Will Cole, leading functional medicine expert and bestselling author of *The Inflammation Spectrum* and *Ketotarian*

"Dr. Caroline Leaf has truly impacted my life, helping me change my life one thought at a time!"

Michelle Williams, singer, actress, author

"During these trying emotional times, Dr. Caroline Leaf offers a helpful and sustainable mind management program that transcends standard self-help. Her book offers a five-step plan to discern and rid ourselves of anxiety and depression to improve our overall health. She is a thought leader to watch."

Dr. Lisa Mosconi, *New York Times*
bestselling author of *The XX Brain*

"Caroline's new book is a lovely chance for us to learn a new modality of healing. The techniques taught in Caroline's work have allowed me to work on myself in new ways that allow me to be more calm, clear, and compassionate."

Jonathan Van Ness, Emmy-nominated television
personality, hairstylist, self-care guru, *New York
Times* bestselling author, and host of the *Getting
Curious with Jonathan Van Ness* podcast

"In *Cleaning Up Your Mental Mess*, Dr. Leaf discusses her search for answers to perplexing questions concerning mental health—and shows how our psyche and emotions release physiological chemicals that negatively affect us cognitively, behaviorally, and emotionally. She sets out to prove that although we must live in a world filled with stressors that keep us in perpetual states of anxiety, we can mitigate these negative effects through self-awareness and simple practices. By understanding the nature of such stressors, which are major contributing factors to mental illness, we will find a remedy stronger than any pharmaceutical—a strategy I call 'mind over matter.'"

Dr. Cindy Trimm, former Bermuda senator,
psychotherapist, author, and humanitarian

"Mental health and illness exist on a continuum. We all move back and forth between the two, sometimes from day to day. It's so important to be aware of our thoughts in order to improve and protect our mental health. Some mental illnesses can be prevented, so efforts to increase our sense of psychological well-being are worthy efforts indeed! Countless readers have come to trust Dr. Leaf's guidance in helping them do just that, and she is at it again with *Cleaning Up Your Mental Mess*. This book is everything we've come to expect from Dr. Leaf's work and more!"

Dr. Anita Phillips, trauma therapist, minister, and mental health advocate

"Dr. Caroline Leaf delivers concrete and scientifically proven answers to the common question, Can I master my mind? If you're ready to take back control in any area of your life, this book will support your journey. A must-read for anyone who is ready for change!"

Vienna Pharaon, licensed marriage and family therapist and founder of Mindful Marriage & Family Therapy

Cleaning Up

YOUR
MENTAL
MESS

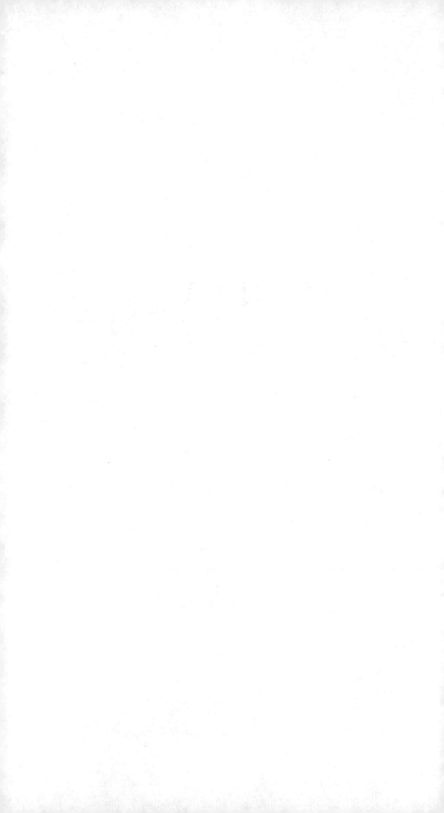

Cleaning Up
YOUR
MENTAL
MESS

5 Simple,
Scientifically Proven Steps
to Reduce Anxiety, Stress, and Toxic Thinking

DR. CAROLINE LEAF

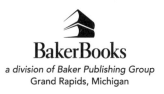

BakerBooks
a division of Baker Publishing Group
Grand Rapids, Michigan

Published by Baker Books
a division of Baker Publishing Group
PO Box 6287, Grand Rapids, MI 49516–6287
www.bakerbooks.com

Printed in the United States of America

Library of Congress Cataloging-in-Publication Data
Names: Leaf, Caroline, 1963– author.
Title: Cleaning up your mental mess : 5 simple, scientifically proven steps to reduce anxiety, stress, and toxic thinking / Dr. Caroline Leaf.
Description: Grand Rapids, Michigan : Baker Books, a division of Baker Publishing Group, [2021]
Identifiers: LCCN 2020042377 | ISBN 9780801093456 (cloth) | ISBN 9781540900401 (paperback)
Subjects: LCSH: Mindfulness-based cognitive therapy. | Mental health. | Mind and body.
Classification: LCC RC489.M55 L43 2021 | DDC 616.89/1425—dc23
LC record available at https://lccn.loc.gov/2020042377

This publication is intended to provide helpful and informative material on the subjects addressed. Readers should consult their personal health professionals before adopting any of the suggestions in this book or drawing inferences from it. The author and publisher expressly disclaim responsibility for any adverse effects arising from the use or application of the information contained in this book.

Some names and identifying details have been changed to protect the privacy of individuals.

The Switch On Your Brain 5-Step Learning Process and the Metacog are registered trademarks of Dr. Caroline Leaf.

22 23 24 25 26 27   13 12 11 10 9 8

This book is dedicated to *you*—to helping you benefit from the research I've done over the past thirty-eight years; the clinical trials recently done with my incredible team of neuroscientists, neurosurgeons, and neurologists; *and* what I have observed in my private practice and around the world.

I want to help you learn how to make the most of your mind and brain, taking your thinking to new heights and transforming your mental landscape through mind-management. This book won't only teach you how to manage your anxiety, depression, stress, and fears but also teach you how to manage your life—from the sad moments to the happy ones to the traumatic ones to the times when you don't even know who you are.

For over three decades, my objective has been to teach individuals, corporations, and institutions what mind-management is and to create easy-to-use and accessible tools that will help people manage their thoughts and lifestyles in more effective ways that bring peace and the ability to live life to its fullest. I hope you'll find these tools helpful in your own life and realize that you have it within yourself to take back control of your mental health and your life!

CONTENTS

We can go three weeks without food, three days without water, three minutes without oxygen—but we can't even go for three seconds without thinking.

PREFACE

Do you ever feel like your brain has just been "switched off"?

Have you ever felt discouraged, unfocused, or overwhelmed?

Are there unhealthy patterns in your life or your family that you just can't seem to break?

Do you start your day exhausted and depressed?

Are you anxious about the future?

Are you haunted by your past?

Do you feel lost and uncertain?

If you answered yes to any of these questions, you're not alone. More and more of us are suffering from anxiety, depression, and burnout.

But this doesn't mean that there's something wrong with you or that you have a mental illness. Anxiety, depression, and post-traumatic stress are all ways of describing natural human responses to adversity and the experiences of life. And we all face adversity in many different ways: challenging events and circumstances are as much a part of modern existence as they were a part of human history.

Calling these mental and emotional responses *diseases* misses the point entirely. Anxiety, depression, burnout, frustration, angst, anger, grief, and so on are emotional and physical warning signals telling us we need to face and deal with something that's happened or is happening in our life. This pain, which is very *real*, is a sign that there's something wrong: you are in a state of disequilibrium. It's not a sign of a defective brain. Your experience doesn't need to be validated by a medical label. Mental health struggles are not your identity. They're normal and need to be addressed, not suppressed, or things will get worse.

Yet this is often what happens. Modern psychological and psychiatric approaches to mental health, particularly the use of drugs like antidepressants and antipsychotics, don't address the complexity of the human mind. Indeed, they haven't reduced the prevalence of mental health issues—major depression, for example, has remained at around 4 percent between 1990 and 2010.

Population studies indicate that something is going terribly wrong: people ages twenty-four to sixty-five are dying eight to fifteen years younger than previous generations from preventable lifestyle diseases. There's a pressing need to change the way we approach health care, including mental health.

We must shift our focus from a symptom-centered approach to one centered around each person's complex story and unique experiences. This is the approach I've taken in this book.

You are uniquely, wonderfully you—your quest for optimal health and well-being should be just as singular as you are.

○ ○ ○ ○

If there is one thing I have learned from my work in this field, it's that we all have to learn how to catch and alter our thoughts and reactions before they become toxic neural networks and habits. How? That's what this book will teach you. In this book, I'll show you *how* to become the interior designer of your mind and brain in five simple steps, using the principles of neuroplasticity. In my clinical practice and research, I developed my Switch On Your

Brain 5-Step Learning Process, and in the years since, I've continued to research and refine these powerful steps toward healthy
mind-management, which I now call the Neurocycle.

In this book, we'll apply the simple, practical, and scientifically
researched and clinically applied 5 Steps of the Neurocycle to such
issues as anxiety, stress, and toxic thinking. We'll also learn how
to build brain and mind health and resilience. You'll find the 5
Steps are sustainable because they'll help you learn how to use
your mind and brain in a way that directs the neuroplasticity of
your brain to your benefit, improving your mental and physical
health in the process.

Mental mess is something we all experience often, and it isn't
something we should be ashamed of. This is my profession, and
I still have to clean up my mind daily—neurocycling is a lifestyle!
The events and circumstances of life aren't going anywhere; people
make a lot of decisions every day that affect us all, and suffering
of some sort for you and your loved ones is inevitable. That said,
I wholeheartedly believe that although events and circumstances
can't be controlled, we can control our *reactions* to these events
and circumstances. This is mind-management in action.

In fact, managing the mind is more than a lifestyle—it's a necessity because you don't even go three seconds without thinking.
If we don't mind-manage our mental mess, our life will feel like
a mess. We can spend lots of money and time on self-help books
and seminars, wellness fads, great teachings, and podcasts. But
all this will simply become nice-to-know information if we can't
apply it—more notches on our belt, more knowledge gathering
dust.

Mind-management through using the 5 Steps of the Neurocycle, on the other hand, can transform all this great information
into *applied* information. When we apply mind-management,
we'll learn how to actually use the advice and information we
gather as we go through life. When we learn how to manage our

mind, we can go from posting inspiring quotes on social media to inspiring others through the way *we actually live* our own life.

o o o o

Part 1 of this book discusses what the mind is, what happens when we don't use our minds properly, and why mind-management using the 5 Steps is the solution to *cleaning up our mental mess*, including the results of my recent research. Part 2 provides my clinically applied and scientifically researched mind-management plan—the Neurocycle.

If our minds are messy, we mess up our lifestyles, and when our lifestyles are messed up, our mental and physical health suffer. The 5 Steps are a way to harness our thinking power—any task that requires thinking can use a neurocycle, which means everything can use a neurocycle because we are always thinking! So, are you ready to begin cleaning up your mental mess?

ACKNOWLEDGMENTS

I want to acknowledge two very special people who have been so instrumental at every level in the writing of this book: my daughters Jessica and Dominique. Dominique is my producer and runs my social media and marketing; Jessica is my research assistant and in-house editor and runs customer service. They have immersed themselves in this project from the creation phase all the way through to the final stages—they were brilliant, supportive, and honest, and I couldn't have done it without them.

A lot of my inspiration, drive, and insight for the work and research I do has also come from my other two children, Jeffrey and Alexandria, who have faced many challenges with resilience.

I also want to acknowledge my husband, Mac, whose endless love is my anchor.

My research team was incredible, and without them this research could not have run like it did, nor could it have been the success that it was. Dr. Robert Turner, neurologist and neuroscientist, approached me a few years ago about the impact of my work with his patients. We ran the research in his neurology clinic, and he oversaw the technical and practical details, along with Charlie Wasserman, his qEEG technologist. Charlie outstandingly handled so many of the practical, on-the-ground details that arise in a research study of this nature. Dr. Jason Littleton, a primary care physician, did a great job advising on the physiological measures and related practicalities. Nick, a phlebotomist, drove tirelessly back and forth between Florida and North Carolina multiple times at each testing point of the study to make sure the bloodwork was done properly. Dr. Darlene Mayo, a neurosurgeon, assisted in the analysis of the results, specifically with the qEEG analysis and graphic displays, and was an incredible help in this complicated process. Elite Research handled the technical side of the proposal and the study, providing statistical analyses and assisting with the preparation for publication. Dr. Rene Paulson, owner of Elite, spent hours walking me through the finer details of the complex statistical analyses and their applications in this study with great insight and wisdom.

And finally, I want to acknowledge the wonderful team at Baker Books, with whom I have worked for eight years! From my amazing editor, Brian Vos, to the teams led by Mark Rice and Lindsey Spoolstra that make things happen—thank you!

PART ONE

THE WHY
AND HOW

Chapter 1

What Happens When We Don't Use Our Minds Correctly

Whatever we plant in our minds and nourish with repetition and emotion will one day become a reality.

EARL NIGHTINGALE

Overview

- If our minds are messed up, our lifestyles are messed up, and when our lifestyles are messed up, our mental and physical health suffer.

- Mind-management is a skill that needs to be *learned and constantly upgraded* as we grow from childhood into adulthood. For every new experience we need a new set of mind-management tools.

- There's no secret quick fix or uniform formula to healing and happiness.

- Feeling guilty because you "failed to think positively enough," "didn't have enough faith," or didn't reach some "ideal" is damaging to your psyche and your physical body.

- For the first time in decades, the trend of people living longer has been *reversed* due to lifestyle-related diseases. Yes, we are in control of our lifestyle choices, but it doesn't seem like we are doing a very good job at this!

- Everything in our society seems to convey the message of "now!" It's almost as if we've entered an era where we have sacrificed the processing of knowledge for the gathering of data.

- Mental distress and ill-health are not new. Humans have always battled mental health issues.

- Mental health has been subsumed into the biomedical model. It has become something we fear and stigmatize, and fear, in itself, is damaging to the brain and body. Our story is not an "it" to be diagnosed and labeled. Depression and anxiety are not labels but rather warning signals.

- We can't control the events and circumstances of life but we can learn to control our reactions, which help us deal with and manage the many challenges we face.

Sometimes it feels like we live in a world characterized by fear. People are fearful about their health, the economy, their jobs, the future, corruption, crime, and their feelings of powerlessness. The cost of this fear is toxic thoughts, toxic stress, anxiety, and depression, which in turn increase our vulnerability to disease. The end result of this fear, anxiety, and illness cycle, if we don't manage it with our minds, is a society dependent on external factors such as painkillers, medications, wellness fads, and skyrocketing health costs to fix us.

But what if there was another way? What if the answer lay inside of you? What if you held the key?

Most people understand the need to live a healthy lifestyle, even if they don't fully understand the impact of their lifestyle choices on disease processes. What many people don't recognize is the need for proper mind-management and how it both supports and sustains a healthy lifestyle.

When our thinking is toxic, it can mess up the stress response, which then starts working against us instead of for us. This, in turn, can make us more vulnerable to disease, which is why many researchers now believe that toxic stress is responsible for up to approximately 90 percent of illness, including heart disease, cancer, and diabetes. Only 5–10 percent of disease is said to come from genetic factors alone.[1]

Why? When an individual is in a toxic thinking state, the release of stress hormones such as cortisol and homocysteine can significantly affect the immune system, cardiovascular system, and neurological system. In fact, excessive stress hormones are so effective at compromising the immune system that physicians therapeutically provide recipients of organ transplants with stress hormones to prevent their immune system from rejecting the foreign implant.

> What many people do not recognize is the need for proper mind-management and how it both supports and sustains a healthy lifestyle.

Despite a more widespread understanding of the importance of healthy lifestyle choices, and many incredible resources out there on making good lifestyle choices, many people lack the necessary mind-management skills they need to apply this knowledge to everyday life. This isn't a one-off thing. Mind-management is a skill that needs to be learned; used all day long, every day; and constantly upgraded as we grow from childhood into adulthood. For every new experience we need a new set of mind-management tools.

Now, before you start panicking and thinking that it's impossible, stop, breathe, and read on. I don't want you to get stuck thinking it's hopeless, that you have caused all your own problems, and that you cannot change. This will only make you feel worse about yourself, and it really isn't the case. You can't blame yourself for something you didn't know—but you can empower yourself and shift into change mode when you learn how to manage your thinking. This is a skill that needs to be learned and constantly upgraded—I do this daily, and will continue to do so until I pass on from this world.

Most of what I share in this book hasn't been taught to you before because it's an area that isn't well understood. We're only beginning to understand mind and consciousness, which is exciting. If we've come this far without good mind-management skills, imagine where we can go when we've learned how to control our thinking.

Mind-Management Must Be a Priority

You are your mind, you are always using your mind, and your mind is always with you. You can go three weeks without food, three days without water, and three minutes without air, but you cannot go three seconds without thinking. So, understanding how the mind works and what mind-management is should be your top priority. Mind-managing your thoughts is a skill that needs to be learned and made into a habit, or, to be more scientifically accurate, *automatized*, much like you learn how to swim or ride a bicycle.

This is what you will be learning in this book. Mind-management is key to the kind of mental peace that sustains us through tough times and happy times. It is the place where you can find your *own* measure of success, instead of comparing yourself to the unrealistic "industry standards" often presented by popular wellness industry and faith movements.

To what and whom are you comparing yourself? Who defines success and says what it looks like for you? *You do*. No one else has the right to define your purpose. We often set ourselves up for failure when we try to copy someone else's healing journey or when we are told the healing process is linear and standard. That's one reason the wellness industry can be so dangerous: it asserts that healing and health come only when certain rules (created by someone else) are followed.

Holding ourselves to a competitive mentality fostered by influencers on social media or by someone offering the elixir of a wellness trend puts impossible demands on our psyche and can be destructive, damaging not only how we see our body image but also how we judge our own worth. Unless we define our wellness within the narrative of accepting that life will always have some mystery, we will drive ourselves crazy with guilt and shame every time our body breaks down or our mind plays up. We'll constantly feel the need to measure up. Instead, we need to validate what we are going through with self-compassion by managing our minds *through* the process of guilt, shame, and sickness, letting these become springboards and not deadweights.

Of course, there's so much great evidence-based information in the fields of positive psychology, the wellness movement, and integrative medicine about the mind-brain connection, and I'm excited that it's talked about now more than it ever has been in my many years of experience. We now know more than we ever have how what we think, feel, and choose directly and indirectly affects our brain and body.

I do, however, have concerns about how some of the research is interpreted, and how it can make some people feel. For example, some people have argued that "Good people don't get sick," or "If I think enough good thoughts or positive affirmations or change my attitude, I will make all the bad stuff go away." This is, often inevitably, followed by a series of toxic guilt or shame thoughts that make us feel worse when our problems don't just disappear. *This is supposed to work! Why isn't it working? What's wrong with me? Why do* they *get it right and not* me?

Feeling guilty or ashamed over not getting healed instantly or feeling bad that you still feel bad or depressed isn't healthy and can make a bad situation worse. There's no secret quick fix or uniform formula to healing and happiness. Let's face it: life is messy.

A better and healthier mindset to have when reading about health and wellness trends is to ask yourself, *Why is this one idea resonating with me?* or *Why am I reading about this and why do I want to know more? What underlying issue am I really trying to address?* and use your answers to gather data and awareness.

I'm not saying that doing one or more popular "healthy" things isn't good for you. I love yoga and organic food, for example. However, using them as a magic formula is guaranteed to disappoint. Feeling guilty because you failed to think positively enough, didn't have "enough" faith, or didn't reach some "ideal" is damaging to your mental psyche and physical body, and the shame and guilt that come with this mindset have a nasty way of spiraling out of control unless they're mind-managed.

> If you don't shape your life, it will be shaped for you.

This toxic idea of "If I just do *x* then *y* will happen" is born out of a distorted view of meritocracy and neurocentricity, where we believe *y* will naturally happen if *x* is done, and *x* is standard for everyone. This belief ignores the impact of individual external (environment, culture, family) and internal (personality, identity) circumstances, setting you up for failure from the start.

This type of thinking can also lead you to internalize failure, as though there's something inherently wrong with you. You may think something like *I have followed the advice or the path or the way; why am I not "fixed?"* But what does "fixed" even mean? Is it some distorted perception of immediate, 100 percent healing? Is it looking a certain way? Or having a certain amount of money? Or perhaps feeling happy all the time? What standard are you using to measure yourself by?

One thing is certain: if you don't shape your life, it will be shaped for you. And to shape your life, you need to know how to shape your mind—you need mind-management.

We Have a Problem

We can't just keep making bad mind-management decisions and think nothing will happen. If we do this, we will be exactly like the moth that keeps coming back to the candle flame and eventually gets burned. Sometimes we're not even aware we're making bad mind-management decisions because it feels so natural or it's just "how other people are doing it."

I believe we live in a day and age where the *mis*management of mind has reached a zenith. For the first time in decades, the trend of people living longer has been *reversed*. People are sicker and dying younger, despite all the advances we have made in medicine and technology. For the first time in modern human history, people are dying younger than their predecessors from— and this is the crazy part—*preventable* lifestyle diseases.[2] Not only are we experiencing pandemics, climate change, and exposure to pollutions harmful to our health, but more and more people are dying from despair.[3]

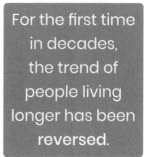

For the first time in decades, the trend of people living longer has been reversed.

Yes, we're in control of our lifestyle choices, but it doesn't seem like we're doing a very good job. Why? Why, with so much good information and technology out there, are we falling so behind?

For the past sixty-plus years, we've spent so much money and time on the physical component of fixing the brain and body that the mind has been thoroughly neglected. Considering the complex and inseparable relationship between our mind and our body, neglecting such an important facet of our humanity can't be done without some sort of cost.

We started noticing this cost in the '80s, but it became glaringly evident in 2014, when federal data showed that for the first time in decades the trend of people living longer has been reversed, with people between the ages of twenty-five and sixty-four the worst affected.[4] Yes, the United States is a pretty well-off country in many ways. However, our mortality rate is going *up*, not down, which doesn't seem to make any sense considering the many advances we've made and the unprecedented amount of knowledge to which we have access. Something serious is going on.

Many people are broken and without hope. It's not surprising that a Brooking's report in October 2019 noted how "deaths of despair" were affecting many sectors of society, particularly in America's heartland.[5] Carol Graham, Brooking Institution's senior fellow, made this eye-opening observation: "The metric that really stands out is not sort of happy, or unhappy. Happy today doesn't matter a whole lot. It's *hope* for the future or lack thereof that's really linked with premature mortality."[6]

More and more research is showing how the absence of hope and the lack of resources to deal with our most basic emotional and physical needs are coming at a great cost. Fear, isolation, pain, purposelessness, despair . . . these are the symptoms of a society that is broken and hurting, and they can lead to an early death not only from suicide but from very real damage to the heart, immune system, GI system, and brain—the entire body goes into states of low-grade inflammation that can increase our vulnerability to disease by up to 75–95 percent when we are in a constant state of turmoil.[7]

Just look at this statement from a 2019 research study:

> A new analysis of more than half a century of federal mortality data . . . found that the increased death rates among people between the

ages of 25–64 extended to all racial and ethnic groups and to sub-
urbs and cities—from suicides, alcohol, drug overdoses and lifestyle
diseases—children are losing parents and the workforce is sicker.[8]

That is not acceptable.

The death rate from chronic debilitating conditions has risen
20.7 percent between 2011 and 2017, and is likely to keep climbing
sharply.[9] The trend is especially bad for middle-aged Americans,
who are more likely to die of cardiovascular disease now than in
2011, reversing decades of improvement.[10]

As a society, we can no longer rest on our laurels and tell ourselves that things are getting better or that we're great. This is
simply not the case, for America or for the wider world. Life expectancy has also been falling in the United Kingdom, for instance,
and the leading causes of death also appear to be lifestyle-related,
including drug use, financial pressure, depression, and isolation.[11]

We can no longer avoid the irony staring us right in the face.
Our social media feeds are full of good advice on how to eat,
great quotations and tips for managing stress, inspirational stories,
wellness trends for longevity and improved life quality—and we're
still getting sick and dying. Suicide rates are on the rise, toxic ad-
dictions are increasing, people are more depressed and anxious
than ever before, and our children are the most medicated of any
generation in history.

What Is Going On?

A large part of the problem is that we've lost much of our ability
to think deeply. We've forgotten the art of deep and focused mind-
management. We want things fast, quick, *now*. We often don't
want to put in the hard work that leads to true change, or we've
never been taught what this kind of work looks like.

The progression into an information era with easy access to endless streams of knowledge has changed how people think, feel, and

make choices. It's almost as if we have entered an era where we've sacrificed the processing of knowledge for the gathering of data. We are, without realizing it, training ourselves to not process but immediately jump to a quick solution and reactive opinion. When no quick fix presents itself, as is often the case with mental health struggles, we become disempowered, feel guilty, and often give up, causing even more damage to our mental and physical health.

We as humans have evolved to *think deeply*, *differently*, and *collectivistically*. When our knowledge isn't being effectively applied, just consumed, our minds become nutritionally starved and can't get from point A to point B. We stop making the jump from knowledge gathering to knowledge application. Gathering information without processing and applying it is counter to how the mind works and how the brain is structured and has a deleterious effect on our mental and physical well-being, creating a mental mess in the mind and a physical mess in the body. As marvelous and necessary as modern technology and all the advances that have come along with it are, we need to learn mind-management skills to use them properly, or we can end up only making more of a mental mess, one that will continue to reduce our quality of life and shorten our life spans.

The Messy Mental Health System

We can see this mess spill over into how we perceive mental health. The management of mental health has become more biomedical and neuroreductionistic over the past fifty years. *Neuroreductionistic* means we have made everything about the physical brain. Your story, including your experiences and the political and socioeconomic environment you live in, has been entirely overlooked and subsumed into a philosophy of "my brain made me do it." Your feelings of depression are because you have a "serotonin imbalance" and "neuropsychiatric brain disease." This neuroreductionistic model does not account for a situation, for example, where you may experience something as detrimental as racism and have been living in fear and anxiety for most of your life because of your skin color. Or, in another example, as a child you were raped by a family member and made to feel it was your fault. Such neuroreductionism ignores the significance of our life experiences and has dominated the world of mental health management for far too long.

According to a recent paper released by biological anthropologists at Washington State University, mental health research is still stuck in a nineteenth-century worldview that was unfortunately given new life in 1980 because of the emergence of the biomedical model of classifying everything by symptoms.[12] This was done in order to reveal underlying neurobiological patterns that would lead to specific solutions, but it hasn't worked. Global rates of depression have been around 4 percent since 1990, while a large meta-analysis of antidepressant trials in 2018 has shown that the large increase of antidepressant use hasn't delivered measurable results.[13] For example, in Australia, usage increased by 352 percent between 1990 and 2002, yet there has been no observed reduction in rates of anxiety, depression, or addiction.

In conflict-affected countries, 1 in 5 people suffer from depression versus 1 in 14 worldwide, indicating that socioeconomic and political issues are important factors in mental health and need to be given far more attention that they currently receive.

Of course, mental distress and ill-health are not new. Humans have always battled them. Life has always been tough, and people have always gone through tough stuff. I don't believe that mental health issues are on the rise, just that they look different in the twenty-first century and we've become far more aware of the pervasive effects of mental distress.

I do, however, believe that the *mismanagement* of mental health issues is on the rise. It's a strange paradox that, even though our understanding of the brain has advanced, our understanding of the mind seems to have gone backward, leading to a very narrow and reductionistic view of the human story. There's been a shift from seeing the mind as having top priority in navigating our complex lives to seeing the mind as a product of our neural networks— and to seeing the sufferings of life as pathologies, which is classic neuroreductionism. This can only spell problems. As philosophers continue to explore the expansiveness of mind, biologists and neuroscientists are trying to map the vastness of the human story onto neural correlates. Many times, it feels like we've progressed two steps forward but taken ten steps back, straitjacketing our mental lives and the complexity of the human experience by focusing solely on our biology and not our stories.

I'm not saying it's been all doom and gloom since the 1800s, nor am I viewing the past with rose-colored glasses. Indeed, modern advances in brain technology have done wonders in the field of neuroscience, helping us better understand the brain. However, when this data is used exclusively to search for the neurobiological correlates of the full human experience, with the lofty objective of mapping a "normal brain," rendering anything outside of this as abnormal and in need of treatment, I believe we're asking the wrong questions and looking for answers in the wrong places.

Weighing the Cost

The current mental healthcare system has largely reduced the source of human pain and suffering to neuropsychiatric brain diseases, with symptoms that need to be suppressed with medication or the conditioning of our thoughts and behaviors. Mental health has been subsumed into the biomedical model. It has become something we fear and stigmatize, and this fear in itself is damaging to the mind, brain, and body.

This perception of mental health has come at great cost. When we only suppress, label, and drug our mental distress instead of embracing, processing, and reconceptualizing the sufferings of life, the pain can become embedded toxic energy in the brain and cells of the body. That can, in turn, affect cognition, damage the brain, and increase our vulnerability. Every system of the body becomes at risk. Over time, this embedded toxic energy can affect how we think, feel, and make decisions, which, in turn, may shorten our life span.

> This neuro-reductionistic perception of mental health has come at great cost.

Neuroreductionism removes a person from their life experiences, making them an "it" that needs to be diagnosed, labeled, and, most likely, treated with psychotropic drugs, which suppress, not cure, the symptoms of mental distress. Mind issues are being treated as if they were a disease like cancer or diabetes, but they're very different. The biomedical model works beautifully for the former but is not the right approach for mental issues like anxiety and depression. These are intrinsically connected to our stories—our place in the world and how we perceive ourselves and our lives. Our story is not an "it" to be diagnosed and labeled. And depression and anxiety are not labels but rather warning signals, telling us that something is going on. As we embrace the warning signals, we find the actual message behind the messenger.

This doesn't mean that mental ill-health doesn't have real, physical effects on the brain and body—of course these are impacted, because the mind is moving through the brain and body and impacting the physiology and neurophysiology right down to the DNA. The mind and the brain are separate but inseparable at the same time. Depression and anxiety are serious and can be debilitating, requiring attention in the form of proper support, understanding, and mind-management. These warning signals affect the 99 percent mind portion—our psyche—*and* the 1 percent physical portion—our brain and body—so they have a 100 percent impact and therefore do not need to be validated with a disease label. They're valid enough in themselves.

There's a significant and well-established association between high psychological distress and early death from things like cancer and cardiovascular disease. The mind-body connection is very real, which we observed in our most recent clinical trial. Even mild depression and anxiety, if left unmanaged, can lead to an estimated 20 percent increase in risk of death from all causes except cancer (which is generally associated with high levels of psychological distress).[14]

Someone suffering from the emotional and physical warning signals of depression and anxiety needs to be noticed and listened to. Their pain, which is very real, needs to be acknowledged, and they need help learning how to problem-solve and manage their minds. They need to tell their story, and we need to listen.

Our current, neuroreductionistic approach to mental health *has not worked*.[15] We need a revolution in mental health care.

In fact, the modern approach to mental health is more than just messy; it can be quite scary. It's very disturbing that psychiatry is the only branch of medicine that can forcibly remove the element of choice from a patient. If you have cancer or diabetes, or any other diagnosed disease, you can refuse treatment—it's your prerogative. But if you get labeled with a mental illness and you refuse medication, you're told that your choice is your disease manifesting. You can quickly lose agency and control of your life. That's not only unethical but also dehumanizing, impeding our fundamental right as human beings to express our pain and have our story told and honored. And it's the reason even the WHO (World Health Organization) is speaking up against this approach, saying it's an attack on the fundamental rights of a person.[16]

The Limitations of Labels

Obviously, a lot of things can go wrong as we go about our lives in vibrant, dynamic human communities. People make choices, and those choices affect us just as much as our choices affect others. We should not, and in fact cannot, medicalize the complexity of the human experience. As much as we love classifications, labels, and systems, we also have to respect that they have their limits—and they have their sting, especially when they follow you into job applications or insurance eligibility or lead you into being too afraid to talk about how you feel because you will be seen as "crazy."

Labels may give a little comfort, but we have to be careful of getting too comfortable, because we may end up avoiding doing the hard work needed to treat the root problem and create sustainable positive change. Don't use labels as a coping mechanism. Rather, use them to better understand where you are and to challenge yourself to overcome what you are dealing with.

Yes, our biology can affect our mental state. For example, a thyroid hormone deficiency can contribute to the onset of depression, and amphetamine abuse can lead to psychosis. However, humans' multifaceted experiences cannot be understood as isolated events. They're intrinsically connected to the whole life history and experience of the individual, and the society in which that individual has grown up.[17] As psychiatrist Joanna Moncrieff explains,

> Whereas thyroid deficiency may provide an adequate explanation of an episode of depression brought on by hypothyroidism, and thyroid hormone will usually provide an adequate treatment, a "normal" episode of depression has to be understood and "treated" in quite a different way, as a human reaction.[18]

It's time for society to start honoring people's stories and what we're going through, not make us feel like there's something wrong with us if we feel sad or depressed or anxious, or that we're abnormal and have failed in some way if we're not happy all the time.

Yes, I do see the appeal a label or pill can have. It is understandable if people need some help or guidance to get to a point where they are able to deal with what is causing their anxiety or depression—they may feel like they are too paralyzed by their pain to even begin to clean up their mental mess. But these solutions are just temporary, and often comes with their own side effects and risks.

Hard work and suffering shape us; adversity builds strength. Suppression makes things worse and will rear its ugly head at some point in our lives, mentally or physically or both, and if we try to rush the process, we can impede our growth and development as human beings. When we accept this truth, we can then begin to focus on how to do the hard work in the most effective way possible. We will spend less energy on constantly trying to make quick fixes work—an exhausting and disheartening endeavor—and more energy on actually addressing and reconceptualizing the root toxic issue.

Of course, it's perfectly okay to say, "This is awful. I don't want to be going through this" when you are in the midst of unbearable emotional and/or physical pain. In fact, I strongly encourage you to do this. It's perfectly okay to ask for help and to get help—this is normal and, once again, I strongly encourage you to do this. However, it's only through the process of embracing and interacting with our pain that we learn how to *manage it* and *get to the other side*. This may take a long time, or it may happen in a few hours or days, but through the process of embracing and reconceptualizing your mental distress, you can learn to mind-manage your way through the tough times. This is something we all need to learn and constantly develop.

Going Forward, Together

Learning how to manage your mind doesn't mean going it alone. We all need all the help we can get as humans in an ever-evolving, hugely complex world, including large doses of gentleness, kindness, and compassion for each other as well as ourselves. We need a new narrative, one where we listen to each other's narratives and problem-solve through them together.

In fact, I strongly encourage you to seek out a support system for your healing journey. The 5 Steps of the Neurocycle method we are going to learn are how you'll get through the day, the week, and the rest of your life. Talking to someone about how these steps are helping you in this journey can give you perspective and provide a sounding board. Humans need this—because as we'll discuss, it's not about you, it's about you in the world. Throughout my years as a therapist, researcher, and mother to four children, I saw that those who sought out or created a support system were the ones who had the most sustainable successes. Don't get drawn into the lie that to ask for help is a weakness. To ask for help takes great strength and is necessary.

At the end of the day, your ultimate focus should be on healing, not boosting your ego by attempting to prove you can go at it alone. A support system can include a family member, a partner, a support group, a therapist, or a church. And, as an added bonus for being open and seeking support, you may just help encourage others to be open and honest as well, setting off a positive cycle that will overtake the toxic cycle of shame, guilt, and stigma often associated with mental health struggles.

That's been the theme of my life's work over the past three decades, including in my most recent clinical trial, which we'll discuss in depth in the next chapters. Indeed, many recent medical and integrative medicine studies show that people who participate in comprehensive mind-management lifestyle programs within strong community settings can learn how to manage their minds and experience significant and meaningful physical and behavioral changes in a number of neurophysiological, physiological, and psychosocial outcomes.

What this essentially means is that although we can't control the events and circumstances of life, we *can learn* to control our reactions, which help us deal with and manage the many challenges we face. This goes beyond mindfulness, positive psychology, and the self-help industry into sustainable life management. And we need each other to make this happen effectively.

> *I am currently on day 5 of your app and found it very helpful with my emotions that are in a hot mess. I am happy to know and realize that for the first time in my life I am learning how to deal with situations and not just putting a Band-Aid on it! The 5 Step program has given me hope again (for the first time in years)!*
>
> MARTIE

Chapter 2

What Is Mind-Management and Why Do We Need It?

> *Any man could, if he were so inclined, be*
> *the sculptor of his own brain.*
>
> Santiago Ramón y Cajal

Overview

- The way we use our minds helps us go from just hearing good advice to living a good life.
- We *all* have to learn how to catch and edit our thoughts and reactions before they trigger toxic chain reactions and become ingrained neural networks, a.k.a. bad habits.
- As we think, the brain literally changes in hundreds of thousands of ways, on cellular, molecular, chemical, genetic, and structural levels—the key is that you can direct this process!
- Any brain, at any age, and no matter what has happened to it, can be made to function at a higher level because of the nature of neuroplasticity.

More and more of us are struggling with anxiety, intrusive thoughts, depression, fear, and toxic ruminations that cause all sorts of mental health problems. In my work, I meet all kinds of people who can't concentrate, can't remember, are burned out, have strained relationships, and are dealing with many kinds of physical issues. The list goes on and on.

So, what's the solution? Should we change our lifestyle? Yes, of course—a healthy lifestyle is important; we should all eat wholesome food, exercise regularly, sleep well and enough, control our stress, limit our screen time, and get outside more, insofar as is possible based on our unique life circumstances. More and more research is showing how many diseases are lifestyle-related (which includes what we think about), so what we choose to do and not do can have important consequences for our mental and physical well-being.

This is even more pressing now, as the decades-long trend of people living longer has been reversed despite the advances we've made in medicine and technology. We *really do* need to change our lifestyle, and thankfully there's no shortage of fantastic advice on how to do so that can be found online, in books, from coaches, and in courses.

> The way we use our minds helps us get from just hearing good advice to actually living a good life.

But how do we get from finding good advice to living the good life? How do we go from reading books, blogs, and social media to actually applying what we learn and transforming it into sustainable and impactful life habits? What is the missing piece? Why do so many people put up with stuff they don't need to, even with all the great resources out there?

Change requires action and application, and both of these are driven by our mind. The state our mind is in affects how it functions, which determines what and how we absorb, apply, and put our thinking into action.

Everything we do begins with a thought. If we want to change anything in our lives, we first have to change our thinking, our *mind*. When we know how to change our mind, we rewire neural networks in the brain that create useful, sustainable, and automatized actions and attitudes—good habits that make us happier and healthier. We get from good advice to a good life with our mind—hence the term *mind-management*.

From Neuroreductionism to Neuroplasticity

I'm a scientist and clinically trained therapist, and my thirty-eight years of clinical work and research have consistently shown me that knowledge of correct, simple, and practical mind-management is the first step to getting anything done. Thinking, feeling, and choosing (also known as our *mind-in-action*) precedes all communication; all we say and do is always preceded by a thought.

The process is so logical that we hardly "think" about it, but it's worth taking the time to do so. It's so obvious that we miss it because we're looking for some elusive, complex key. Our mind is staring us in the face, and mind-management is therefore a critical skill we need to learn. As I will show you in this book, if our mind isn't managed, everything downstream will be chaos—a mental mess produces a messy life.

Unfortunately, in our era we have focused so much on the biology of the brain that we have forgotten about the mind. Perhaps you didn't even know they were two different things. Indeed, if you just read a handful of neuroscientific articles at random, you would think we're preprogrammed mechanical brains walking around and occasionally malfunctioning.

Yes, this is a caricature, but it isn't far from the truth. Many professionals and researchers pay attention only to the symptoms of how someone feels, not *why* they feel, because it's a lot easier to deal with one-dimensional symptoms than multidimensional causes, especially as visits to the doctor become shorter and pre-scribing a pill becomes easier. Even people in the medical sys-tem complain how bad it has become. Despite their vast medical knowledge, they are suffering from high rates of mental health issues themselves because they do not understand the mind and how to heal it. It is estimated that one doctor in the United States commits suicide every day.[1] This is one of the main reasons I train physicians on the importance of the mind, correct mind-management, how to manage their mental health, and how to help their patients with mental health issues.

Thankfully, there are signs that things are changing. More and more people are beginning to recognize that there's more to self-transformation than a pill or a program. Sustainable and attain-able change means getting your mind in order *first*, not waiting for that job promotion, losing that weight, or going to that exercise class four times a week. It all starts in the mind.

Every moment of managing your mind is selective. It's just as easy to generate negative changes as it is to generate positive changes in the brain—this is called the *plastic paradox*. The abil-ity of the brain to change, or *neuroplasticity*, can occur in a good or bad direction—the point is that your brain is always changing. The mind is the force that drives neuroplasticity; this is why I say the mind changes the brain, and also why we need to take control of the process like a sailor mastering the wind—or we will be blown any which way.

This book will teach you how to be a neuroplastician—or in other words to become your own mind-surgeon (but without all the blood!). I'll explain the difference between the mind and the brain, what a thought is and how we build thoughts with our mind, how we control our thoughts with our mind, and how we detox our mind and brain *using our mind*.

You can learn a simple but highly effective and scientific mind-management plan—the Neurocycle—to control the "everyday crazy" in your life, because let's face it, life is a little crazy sometimes. Learning the skill of mind-management will help you truly change your lifestyle, define your story, navigate any mental or physical obstacles you face, and help those around you who may be struggling as well.

Mind-in-Action

How we react or respond to various life situations and the world around us is called *mind-in-action*. The mind-in-action is how you uniquely think, feel, and choose. This changes the way our brain functions, our biochemistry, and the genes associated with mental and physical health, which is why mind-management is essential—and a skill to be learned. You, with your mind that is always in action, are the change agent. Correct mind-management means responding in a way that builds healthy neural networks rather than simply reacting and building toxic neural networks. You can be a "first responder" in every and all situations.

We *all* have to learn how to catch and edit our thoughts and reactions before they trigger toxic chain reactions and become ingrained neural networks, a.k.a. bad habits. We also have to learn how to embrace, process, and reconceptualize thoughts that have already become enmeshed in the networks of our minds as trauma and negative thinking patterns. This is a lifelong journey, a lifestyle, and one that's well worth the effort. Just like cleaning your home, washing the car, bathing the dog, or brushing your teeth, a little bit of daily work goes a long way toward helping you feel clean, refreshed, and healthy.

And *now* is the time to do this. When I started my research back in the '80s, many people thought the brain couldn't change—if something was wrong, you were just taught to compensate. When

> We all have to learn how to catch and edit our thoughts and reactions.

I began investigating how deliberate and intentional mind-directed thinking could change behaviors, many of my peers called my ideas ridiculous until I started publishing my results. In one area of my research, I found that if someone had a language, communication, intellectual, or social disability from a trauma or traumatic brain injury (TBI), they could improve their cognitive, intellectual, and social functioning by 35 to 75 percent through directed and deliberate deep-thinking techniques.

That's why I've spent my career trying to understand the mind and developing different ways of using the mind to learn new information, build memory, and manage emotions and mental health.

Resilience

The resilience of the human mind has continually surprised me over the years. Traveling to various countries and working and doing my research in different communities has taught me so much—things I could have never learned in a research lab. Each moment, each story, each person has been another epiphany.

I've seen former addicts turn into community leaders and mobilize change when they learned what they could do with their minds. I've seen teachers with one textbook educating hundreds of children, transforming their classrooms into a wall-to-wall curriculum using the 5-Step learning process and the Metacog writing system I developed (see appendix B). I've seen TBI patients go from being reduced intellectually to a second-grade level to finishing school and getting a university degree. I've seen people battling with autism learn how to manage their emotions. I've seen patients with Alzheimer's slow down cognitive decline. I've seen countless children and adults with learning disabilities learn how to learn. And I've seen parents, students, and grandparents sitting under trees helping each other learn to manage their trauma and anxieties.

All these experiences have been both awe-inspiring and humbling. They've motivated me, kindling my desire to learn more and more about the mind and how I can help people recognize their intrinsic, magnificent potential.

My life's mission, and why I do what I do, is to help people realize how much power they have in themselves to heal their minds, brains, and bodies. I've dedicated my life to finding out how to make mental health care and knowledge easily applicable, affordable, and accessible to everyone. You may not have access to a therapist, but you do have something more powerful: your mind.

> You're not a broken or defective brain.

You're not a broken or defective brain. You never have to settle or just learn to compensate. There are many things you can and should do that can alter, change, slow down, and even reverse the current state of your brain and body. These things are mind-driven: they're the result of your choices, which are the result of your feelings, which are the result of your thinking. This is the mind-in-action.

Quantum Theory

Quantum theory demonstrates the importance of the mind-in-action. *Quantum* means "energy," and it's a very powerful way of explaining the energy associated with the mind, learning, and memory, alongside neuroscience and neuropsychology. For this reason, I've incorporated it into the development of my theory, The Geodesic Information Processing Theory (see appendix A), to explain how the mind-brain connection works and the necessity of mind-management.

Oxford philosopher and theologian Keith Ward calls quantum physics "the most accurate model ever developed to understand the deepest things."[2] Two of these "deepest things" are how we uniquely think as human beings and what our purpose on this earth is.

What is human consciousness—or mind—and why do we have it? Why and how do we think? Quantum physics gives us a way of describing the powerful energy of human consciousness by showing us how incredible our mind is. It provides a scientific theory that describes our ability to choose, and thus our ability to transform our brain, body, and the world around us. It highlights the importance of thinking and how we're all brilliantly, wonderfully unique. Quantum physics points at something we all sense intuitively: that our conscious thoughts have the power to affect our actions. This book will teach you the mental precision needed to harness this power.

This all sounds nice, but what does quantum physics and all this mind talk have to do with your daily life? Well, have you ever asked yourself, *Who is this person I've become?* or *What can I do that could help me change and or manage my problems? Am I actually happy and at peace? How do my thoughts, feelings, and choices impact the world around me?*

Searching for these answers often goes two ways. Perhaps you believe you're a prepackaged, preprogrammed genetic avatar. The fates have decided what will happen to you—there's no fighting it. Or you believe you have some level of influence over the quality of your life, perhaps through that elusive magic elixir, that exercise regimen, that new diet, or that meditation or breathwork you just did. Or maybe you do all these things and just hope for the best—because they're healthy and good for you and must do something, right?

And you may feel good for a few hours, but what happens when things aren't going so well? What do you do when your spouse walks mud into the carpet, that person you can't stand at work sends you a nasty email, or your best friend has a breakdown?

The 5-Step Neurocycle

Good mind-management skills can take you beyond healthy but short-lived mindfulness practices, such as meditation, which help in the moment to calm and prepare the brain but often don't address the main issues behind your thinking. Meditation may bring awareness, but what do you do with that awareness? Awareness, not managed correctly, can do more harm than good. In fact, my research, which I describe in upcoming chapters, shows that awareness without management skills or techniques adversely affects our mental and physical health. When you start understanding how your mind works and how to use the mind-management Neurocycle to address this awareness and change your brain, you create sustainable changes by affecting the root of your issues rather than just their symptoms. You move beyond a "fate versus me" sense of reality. You recognize that life can be tough and bad things happen, but you have built the scaffolding needed to maintain your grounding amid the storm.

This doesn't mean we won't get upset, angry, unhappy, or irritated. We all take some weathering, but we can know how to deal with these emotions and feelings when we experience them *in a scientific way that will actually change the brain and increase our resilience*. That's how these things don't throw us out of joint for days or even weeks. And that's how they don't take over our life.

Let me give you an example. (This is an example of relationships, but the same 5 Steps can be used in any circumstance or situation.) Say you're treated really badly by someone you trust. Now the old you would have immediately sent some nasty texts, perhaps a few good riddance one-liners, and then cried and swore at any living thing that crossed your path. But the new, mind-managed, quantum superhero you instead goes immediately through the different phases of mind-management, the 5 Steps of the Neurocycle method we will discuss in depth in part 2 of this book.

First, you prep that amazing brain of yours, and this is where mindfulness, meditation, breathwork, tapping, and so on are essential. You can do some breathwork (my favorite, because of its scientific base and effectiveness, is the Wim Hof method)[3] or something similar. This is a simple, mind-driven action that prepares your mind and optimizes your brain and body, allowing you to calm down enough to react in the most favorable way. Next, you go *beyond* the mindfulness your preparation has created *into directed neuroplasticity* through the 5 Steps:

1. **Gather.** *Read, listen, and watch what you are thinking and how you are feeling.* Remind yourself that this person often uses their actions and words as a cry for help and this is a sign that they're trying to make sense of what is happening to them, but they don't know how to correctly verbalize their needs or pain. It can be helpful to remember that often how people treat you is a projection of their own turmoil and state of mind. Embrace and accept the fact that you feel hurt or frustrated; don't suppress your emotions or feel guilty for them. But recognize that these emotions will pass. They don't have to define your next actions or thoughts.

2. **Reflect.** *Ask, answer, discuss this with yourself.* Try to find the deeper meaning behind their words and actions. What are they going through? How are they hurting? What's making them react in this way? Don't absorb their negative energy and make it part of you or part of your brain. Stop, stand outside of yourself, and choose to objectify the situation.

3. **Write.** *Journal and organize your thoughts.* Put what you're going through down in your journal or the notes section on your laptop or smartphone, whatever works for you. This will help you organize your thoughts, which will release the emotional sting of your pain—get it out of your body instead of keeping it in. Write what they said and your response, or how you would like to respond.

4. **Recheck**. *Reanalyze and examine what you have written down*. Talk to someone else to get a wider perspective on the situation and your planned response.

5. **Active Reach**. *Apply what you have learned in some tangible way*. Once you've calmed down, reach out in love and ask them what you can do. Even if this just means listening to them as they express their emotions.

The Mind

The most fundamental definition of mind is how you *think, feel, and choose*, which is what you were doing in the example 5-Step Neurocycle process above. The mind works through the brain: the brain is the physical organ that filters and responds to the mind.

Based on my research and clinical experience, I believe that the mind is the biggest part of us, the 90 to 99 percent of who we are. There's compelling evidence showing that mind-in-action, our thinking, feeling, and choosing that includes paying attention to something, building memory in a deliberate way, predicting something, and expecting an event affects our cortical plasticity (neuroplasticity). This means that as you think, feel, and choose, you will expect and believe, and in doing so you're reshaping your mental landscape—your brain is responding to your mind.

These changes happen throughout the brain. The neuroplasticity of the brain isn't isolated to a single system; the directed mind-management of the Neurocycle remodels entire systems and networks in the brain. It even empowers under-functioning brains, drives neurologically impaired brains, and can have a notable corrective effect in traumatized brains. The brain is not hard-wired or stuck; it's

> Our mind is not just a byproduct of our brain.

soft-wired, which essentially means it responds to what we think, feel, and choose—and what we eat, what we put into and onto our body, and how we move our body. Our mind is not just a by-product of our brain.

Now, just imagine using your mind and taking advantage of this neuroplasticity in a way that improves your brain function to the point where you have a plan in place to deal with the challenges of life, preventing them from compromising your happiness and therefore decreasing your vulnerability to disease. Well, by understanding how your mind works and how to use the 5 Steps, you're essentially using the full power of neuroplasticity to your advantage to clean up your mental mess!

Mind-management doesn't just change your brain state, or the way you feel in the moment. It also boosts your cognitive resilience over time because you're facilitating an environment that's healthy for your brain. A strong mind means a strong brain and vice versa in a feedback loop, which gives you the mental strength to face adversity and helps you cope from day to day. It guides you in the midst of a crisis and gives you the determination to wade through times of uncertainty and suffering. It makes you look inward, compelling you to examine, wonder, ask, and deal with what's holding you back.

Directed Neuroplasticity

The 5 Steps provide a mind-management process that takes you from being a bystander watching the car crash to being a first responder and, eventually, to preventing the car crash in the first place. In the same way that nausea, sweating, and going to the bathroom free the body from toxic matter, embracing our mental pain through mind-management, and accepting the uncertainty that comes along with it, helps free us from our toxic experiences, whether a bad habit we've developed over time or a trauma from our past. It may be a little uncomfortable at first, and we may feel some pressure and pain, but we will feel a million times better afterward. With mind-management, even the most fundamental problems can be addressed—as you will see in part 2 of this book.

As we think, the brain literally changes in hundreds of thousands of ways on cellular, molecular, chemical, genetic, and structural levels. More and more research is being published on a daily basis showing how every functional, chemical, and physical feature of the brain can be and is transformed as we use our mind. *The key is that you can direct this process.* You don't have to just let life shift and shape what is between your ears. You don't have to just absorb everything you see and hear.

As we train ourselves in deliberate mind-management, we drive many of the thousands of elemental processes that define the state of our brain function. Indeed, changes in the brain just from learning one new skill are massive; the brain, under the direction of the mind, literally remodels its neurological coding in the dendrites, which are the branches on the tops of neurons that hold our thoughts and memories.

One of the first things you have to start doing to manage your mind is to train the brain to *learn how to learn* in an organized and meaningful way. This is the science of brain-building, which starts when you're a baby and continues throughout your life. However, to take full advantage of this process, the skill of mind-management needs to be developed and enhanced.

Brain-building, like exercising the body, is a core aspect of growing and sustaining your mental and brain health. Each one of us is bursting with potential: with skills, abilities, information, and ideas waiting to be imagined and realized. The 5 Steps of the Neurocycle will help you determine what you need to release this potential, to sustain and grow your neuroplastic brain, *and* to harness all your unmet potential to make necessary lifestyle changes and affect your world for the better. This is not just for some people—mind-management is for everyone. Everyone can learn and grow their brain. Brain-building is as essential to mental and physical health as eating and breathing, which is why it is addressed first in part 2. Detoxing trauma and habits are so much easier if brain-building is incorporated into your lifestyle!

Clinical Trial

I've seen this throughout scientific literature and also in my own most recent clinical trials. From January through December 2019, I conducted two research studies: a validation study (which measures the accuracy of a scale) on the Leaf Mind-Management Scale (LMM), which I developed and have used over many years in my clinical practice, and a random controlled and double-blind clinical trial to evaluate the importance of mind-management using the updated, researched, and clinically applied 5-Step process.

I conducted this research in a US neurology practice with a world-renowned team of doctors and researchers. Indeed, the idea for this research began when a neurologist and friend approached me with a problem: his patients were positively responding to neurofeedback therapy but weren't always carrying this effect over into their daily life. Neurofeedback therapy is "also known as EEG (electroencephalogram) biofeedback . . . a therapeutic intervention that provides immediate feedback from a computer-based program that assesses a client's brain wave activity."[4]

Something more was needed. How did they take the step from a good neurofeedback session to a good life? This particular doctor had started using the 5-Step program as described in my book *Switch On Your Brain* in his practice and found quite dramatic changes in himself and his patients that *lasted* over time—changes evidenced not only in their brain waves as seen on the qEEG (the digital mathematical analysis of EEG data)[5] but also in their actual lifestyles.

I had seen this in my practice and research for years, and in the work I do, so he and I decided to see if these changes could be replicated in a controlled study and validation trial on the updated version of the 5 Steps, the Neurocycle. So, over several months, my research team and I conducted a clinical trial with a group of people from different backgrounds and ages, and we found that people can learn to self-regulate their minds and take advantage of the neuroplasticity of their brains to rework their neural circuitry in a positive direction in 63-day cycles—not twenty-one days, though that number is often touted as how long it takes to form a habit. We did this by using the Neurocycle to manage a variety of mental and physical states, which helped the subjects in the clinical trial form new mental habits and manage their reactions to the circumstances of life.

This validation study and clinical trial, along with an increasing number of studies in neuroimaging literature, highlight the importance of appropriate mind-management training and self-regulation. The bottom line is this: we cannot improve our lifestyle until we learn how to manage our thinking.

This is incredibly *empowering*. The subjects in our experimental group, using our app, went from awareness of their toxic thinking and lack of mind-management to reconceptualizing these mindsets into a new way of seeing themselves and the world around them. This was evident not only in their personal narratives but also on my neuropsychological LMM scale and in various other clinical psychological scales we used to measure participants' brain activity and physiology. We even saw significant changes in the health of their immune system, blood, cells, and DNA.

> We cannot effectively improve our lifestyle or hope the changes will be sustainable until we learn how to manage our thinking.

During these trials, we examined the mind-body interaction and how this changed as our subjects learned how to manage their mental mess using the app. There was an upward trend across all measures in the experimental group versus the control group, as their ability to manage their minds was vastly improved, which helped reduce their anxiety, depression, and mental ill-health by up to 81 percent. The subjects in the experimental group were using their minds (their ability to manage their thoughts, feelings, and choices) to take advantage of the neuroplasticity of their brains and rework and regenerate their neural circuitry. In sixty-three days, they built healthy new thinking habits and improved their overall well-being—and this was sustained after six months and carried over positively into other areas of their life.

As we dig deeper into the results of my research, you'll see how managing your mind is not only doable but also beneficial and can positively affect your mind health, brain health, blood physiology, and even cellular and heart health. Learning to manage your mind through using the 5 Steps of the Neurocycle can help you manage mental distress like depression, anxiety, toxic stress, and intrusive thoughts, help you improve your immunity and cell health, and help protect against cognitive decline and the dementias.

In chapter 4, where we really dig into the science of my research, you'll find sections titled "How Does This Help You?" that give you easy, scientific mind-management tips to motivate you. As a bonus, if you really dig through this science chapter and try to understand it, it will challenge your mind, which will increase your intelligence, grow your brain, and develop your resilience. I've also included some amazing head maps and graphs that show you what anxiety, depression, and chaotic thinking do to your brain, as well as how your brain changes positively as you manage your mind.

In our clinical trial, we observed that people can rewire and regenerate dysfunctional brain networks and physiology from toxic thoughts, altering them with their minds. We have incredibly powerful minds—we have within ourselves the path to true and lasting success.

This path to empowerment over our mental health and well-being doesn't lie in just pills or devices: it's in our own ability to guide and direct changes in our brain. Can you imagine a world where the way we use our minds is seen as an "anxiolytic" and "antidepressant" too? Well, that day is here.

This is not "self-help." This is a scientifically proven and clinically applied *sustainable* mind-management program that has been tried, tested, and proven over thirty-plus years, a way of thinking that makes the best of mindfulness and self-help.

> This is not "self-help." This is a scientifically proven and clinically applied sustainable mind-management program that has been tried, tested, and proven.

As you learn to operate *beyond mindfulness*, you add qualitative understanding and meaningfulness to your lived experience. You go beyond being aware in the *now* moment to *managing* your thought life, gaining the skills to build knowledge, and learning how to apply that knowledge.

The 5 Steps for mind-management presented in this book will help you proactively build mind and brain health, as well as maintain good thinking habits and a good lifestyle, helping you use your memory banks of knowledge in ways that boost and protect your brain health and mental health. Each of the 5 Steps has been meticulously and neuroscientifically researched and is designed to stimulate the highest level of functional response in the brain in the most efficient way possible in order to guarantee healthy thoughts, healthy brain tissue, and good energy flow, all of which contribute to that deeply seated sense of peace that comes with *controlling your reactions* to life.

Learning how to manage your mind will help you clean up your mental mess and live your best life, regardless of your circumstances.

> *I experienced sexual abuse when I was five years old by a relative, and I suppressed all of it, unintentionally, until I was ultimately pushed over the edge by a trigger right after I got married to my husband. I am on day 14 of your 5 Step program, and I am seeing healing like I never thought possible. I have been inspired to help others who went though the same sort of thing I did, and am thinking about going back to school to further my education and become a child trauma therapist.*

> KRISTEN

Chapter 3

Why the Neurocycle Is the Solution to Cleaning Up Your Mental Mess

Nothing in life is to be feared, it is only to be understood. Now is the time to understand more, so that we may fear less.

MARIE CURIE

Overview

- Simple mind-management tools for personal use—to address and ameliorate such warning signals as anxiety, depression, toxic thinking, inability to concentrate, irritability, exhaustion, and burnout before they take over someone's mind and life—can help innumerable persons of all ages experience improved mental and physical health and well-being.

- Our research contributes to the larger body of research that shows how feeling more self-regulated and in control of life can lead to better mental health, because you're no longer just a bystander. When you learn how to clean up your mental mess, you become a "first responder" and decision maker in your life.

> • Empowerment is that missing link that gets you from point A, hearing or reading good advice, to point B, actually applying it in a meaningful and sustainable way.

We can no longer ignore the rise of anxiety, depression, anger, frustration, toxic stress, and burnout in people of all ages in our society. We need to address it head-on. Stressors and changes in life situations trigger responses and changes in our biochemistry, brain function, and genetics, which not only affect our health but can also be passed on through generations, which is known as *epigenetics*. And so, mind-management is both a matter of how we want to live today and how we want our children to live in the future.

As I mentioned in chapter 1, many current mental health strategies, including pharmaceuticals and interventions with medical devices, have not helped us eradicate or even fully manage the devastating mental health conditions that plague our society. Nearly eight hundred thousand people die by suicide in the world each year, which is roughly one death every forty seconds. Suicide is the second leading cause of death in the world for those ages fifteen to twenty-four. Unmanaged depression is the leading cause of disability worldwide.[1]

Simple mind-management tools for personal use—to address and ameliorate such warning signals as anxiety, depression, toxic thinking, inability to concentrate, irritability, exhaustion, and burnout before they take over someone's mind and life—could help innumerable persons of all ages experience improved mental and physical health and well-being.

To that end, I have developed a simple 5-Step mind-management process, called the Neurocycle, based on my research over the past thirty years and the latest brain science, to help you manage your mind and overcome issues like depression, anxiety, and burnout, which can come from chronic recurrent stress, acute sudden stress, trauma, identity issues, isolation, disrupted sleep patterns, lack of exercise, poor diet, and so on, as well as help you to build brain health and mental resilience.

This 5-Step process is based on the science of thought, specifically how we form thoughts with our mind. It goes beyond self-help and mindfulness exercises, taking them to another level by extending them into a sustainable mind-management strategy—the Neurocycle. These steps were developed as a response to my patients' need for a simple yet sustainable and effective way to manage their chronic and acute mental health issues, as well as to build their brain health and resilience. I prioritized making them simple but still highly effective, because when you are already overwhelmed with a chaotic mind, the last thing you want is a bunch of complex techniques!

True personal transformation requires mind-management to rewire and regenerate neural pathways and create new habits. Eventually, as we manage our thinking, the entire state of the brain as well as the cellular and biochemical structures shift and establish a new, healthy level of balance in the mind, brain, and body.

Is the Neurocycle a Solution to Cleaning Up the Mental Mess?

In our clinical trial, two groups of subjects were studied to find out if the updated Neurocycle really is an effective solution to cleaning up the mental mess. The first group, called the *experimental group*, consisted of six subjects trained to use the Neurocycle app, which incorporates the updated, researched, and clinically applied 5 Steps of the Neurocycle method.[2] The experimental group was asked to choose a specific toxic thought to work on overcoming during the clinical trial and to independently use the app daily for sixty-three days as a mind-management tool to help them overcome and rewire (or reconceptualize) a toxic thought or mindset that was disturbing their mental well-being.

The second group of subjects, called the *control group*, was not given instructions to choose a toxic thought to work on, and was *not* given the app to use during the course of the study.

For all subjects, we studied their neuroscientific (qEEG), psychosocial (psychological scales and narratives), neurophysiological (blood), and cellular (telomeres) measures at day 1, before beginning the study, at day 21, and at day 63 of the trial. We then compared the results between the control and experimental groups. On days 7, 14, and 42, and at 6 months, additional psychosocial measures were done, which included their narrative, the Leaf Mind-Management Scale (LMM), and the other psychological measures but not bloodwork or qEEGs. The six-month mark was a follow-up to evaluate the sustainability of the results; that is, how effective mind-management techniques are in the long run.

> Eventually, as we manage our thinking, the entire state of the brain and the cellular structure shifts and establishes a new, healthy level of balance in the mind, brain, and body.

The results were very exciting, and I'm thrilled to share them with you. I truly believe they can change your life for the better, because when you learn how powerful your mind is and how to manage it, there's no going back.

Throughout our research trial, the experimental group saw *significantly positive* changes at a cellular level, which is based on changes in telomeres (the caps on chromosomes that determine the health of the cells), *significantly positive* changes in electrical activity in the brain (based on qEEG-measured changes in the brain), *significantly positive* changes in psychosocial profiling (based on changes in psychological scales and narratives), and *significantly positive* changes in the blood tests (including changed cortisol and homocysteine levels, which show how the body is responding to stress and inflammation). Our results also indicate that there were positive changes in the nonconscious mind (qEEG), conscious mind (LMM), body (telomeres and blood), and whole person (narrative).

This means that the subjects in the experimental group, by using the 5 Steps in the app, *significantly* improved their mental health, brain health, blood physiology, and cellular health—and so can you.

Empowerment Is a Missing Link to Cleaning Up the Mental Mess

In this clinical trial, one of the psychological measures studied was the LMM (Leaf Mind-Management Scale). This tool measures factors such as self-regulation, awareness, sense of autonomy, number of toxic thoughts and amount of toxic stress, perceived barriers, and felt degree of empowerment. The experimental group subjects, those who used the app daily, self-reported that they felt they were set on a pathway to empowerment throughout the study. As we examined the study results, we identified that this was achieved by increasing their autonomy and feeling of control.

This research contributes to the larger body of research that shows how feeling more self-regulated and in control of life can lead to better mental health, because you're no longer just a bystander but now a "first responder" and decision maker in your life.

Autonomy ultimately increased subjects' hope, and the 5 Steps also increased their feelings of being more in control over life and health and less subject to uncertainty. This, in turn, led to increased awareness of and ability to deal with their toxic thoughts, which helped them control toxic stress and change their perspective about how they were looking at the world. They started seeing challenges and barriers as opportunities and had more overall life satisfaction. The Neurocycle literally provided a pathway to empowerment.

This pathway is critical to making the difficult changes needed to heal yourself mentally and physically. It increases resilience in the brain and mind and pain tolerance. Just think of a tough workout routine you have done in the past. What helped you complete it despite the mental and physical strain? Most likely it was a motivating coach or partner who helped you feel capable of change. In this clinical trial, we saw that the mind-management process *scientifically increased the subjects' sense of empowerment*, therefore increasing their emotional and stress resilience.

Empowerment is that missing link that gets you from point A, hearing or reading good advice, to point B, actually applying it in a meaningful and sustainable way.

Path to Empowerment

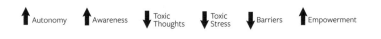

The pathway to empowerment. As we gain increased autonomy by taking control of our mental health, we become more aware of both our issues and our capacity to deal with toxic thoughts and control toxic stress. When we change our perspective, we see opportunities instead of barriers. This process leads us to become more empowered so we can control our lives by controlling our minds.

Depression and Anxiety Are Reduced by 81 Percent Using the Neurocycle

Preliminary results from our trial also demonstrated a significant reduction in depression and anxiety, through using the Neurocycle method for mind-management, by up to 81 percent in the experimental group compared with the control group. We saw these significant changes in many of the measures studied, particularly when analyzing qEEG results. qEEG, or *quantitative electroencephalography*, involves placing electrodes on the scalp to measure the electrical activity inside the brain. Typically, qEEG data are viewed overlaid onto a "map" of the head, so we can see which areas of the brain have more or less electrical activity (prefrontal cortex [PFC], amygdala, hippocampus), and which brain frequencies (delta, theta, alpha, beta, and gamma) are more predominant in different areas of the brain.

The patterns we see on qEEG head maps can help tell us if someone is feeling depressed, anxious, or burnt out; is not managing toxic stress; or feels their identity is being affected; and so on. They can also show when a person is feeling back in control of their mind and is processing issues and learning new ways of thinking. Below is a table summarizing these wave frequencies and what they tell us.

TABLE 1. The Five Wave Frequencies in the Brain

Delta (0–4hz)	*Deep nREM sleep, repair, complex problem-solving.* High amplitudes of delta are also found in people who are in touch with the nonlocal spiritual mind even when they're wide awake, such as the brains of meditators, intuitives, and healers.
Theta (4–8hz)	*Creativity, insight, healing, light sleep, vivid dreams (REM sleep).* The dominant frequency in healing, high creative states, remembering emotional experiences (good and bad), memory retrieval, and encoding. Theta frequency activity is increased, especially at frontal sites, during activities that require attention or short-term memory such as mental arithmetic and working memory load tasks. Information-sharing behavior might be associated with higher theta amplitudes, particularly at frontal sites, since this behavior demands engagement of higher cognitive processes. Theta activates during self-regulation.
Alpha (8–12hz)	*An optimal state of relaxation and alertness, bridging between the conscious and nonconscious mind, which brings peacefulness and readiness and aids meditation.* Alpha connects the higher frequencies—the thinking mind of beta and the associative mind of gamma—with the two lowest-frequency brain waves.

Beta (12–15hz)	*Processing, being alert and attentive, working through something challenging, focusing, having sustained attention.* This is known as "workhorse energy" and represents our normal waking state of consciousness when our attention is directed at something. This is when we do cognitive tasks and engage with the outside world in an active state of learning.
High Beta (15–40hz)	*Bursts of high beta are the signature brain waves of intensity and indicate paying attention and making a choice as the wave collapses in a figurative and quantum sense.* Continual crashes suggest anxiety, frustration, or being under stress. Amplitude of high beta increases with stress, and large flares occur when we experience anger, guilt, shame, and blame. This shuts down the brain regions that handle rational thinking, decision-making, memory, and objective evaluation. Blood flow to the prefrontal cortex, the "logical analytical" part of the brain, can be reduced by up to 80 percent. Starved of oxygen and nutrients, the brain's ability to think clearly can plummet.
Gamma (40–200hz)	*Flows from the front to the back of the brain at forty times a second and contributes to the subjective experience of consciousness, highlighting introspection, high-level learning, deep intellectual function, association and creative inspiration, and the integration of information from different parts of the brain in a compassionate and caring state.* Gamma is also associated with retrieval and encoding.

As the subjects in the experimental group started managing their minds using the Neurocycle, we saw positive changes in the energy patterns in the brain. A general pattern of bursts of high beta and alpha balancing between the left and right hemispheres began to emerge, creating a bridge between the conscious and nonconscious mind over the prefrontal cortex as the subjects chose to deliberately and consciously embrace and focus on finding the cause of the signals of depression or anxiety or both that they were feeling and to reconceptualize these patterns. In other words, they were learning how to make the anxiety and depression work for them and not against them.

These results also showed higher beta and theta activity over the hippocampus (memory) and amygdala (emotional perceptions) as subjects recalled a toxic thought by paying attention to the emotional and physical warning signals. We then observed a shift in beta and gamma activity back to the prefrontal cortex as subjects consciously reflected on this information. This pattern highlights the interaction that happens between the conscious and nonconscious mind as we think deeply. This is a good pattern we want to see in our brain because it reflects mind-management developing.

Below is a table summarizing the brain structures we'll refer to in this book.

TABLE 2. Brain Structures

Brain Structure	Description
Prefrontal Cortex (PFC)	Active when we are awake and consciously thinking, feeling, and making choices, and very active when we are intentional and deliberate about doing so.
Dorsolateral Prefrontal Cortex (DLPFC)	An area in the PFC specifically active when switching attention, working memory, maintaining abstract rules, and inhibiting inappropriate responses.
Amygdala	Responds to emotional perceptions, like a library holding the emotional feelings attached to memories.
Hippocampus	Active when we convert short-term memory to long-term memory.

New Thoughts and New Habits—Evidence of Neuroplasticity

Our experimental group also showed evidence of neuroplasticity. We observed new thoughts with their memories forming, which correlated with a reported improvement in the management of the symptoms of depression and anxiety, including fewer toxic thoughts and less toxic stress, and an improved sense of life satisfaction and well-being, as measured in both the Leaf Mind-Management Scale (LMM) and the narrative reports. Subjects were essentially shifting the way the brain processed information and changing the structures of the brain in a positive direction. That is *directed neuroplasticity*, growing health into the brain. The brain can be intentionally changed by the mind—that is, our thinking, feeling, and choosing.

In fact, in the qEEG results, we observed new neural networks being formed in the brain by day 21—seen as gamma peaks, which are like the tops of waves—in the experimental subjects but not in the control subjects. Gamma peaks and changes in gamma indicate learning is taking place, which means new thoughts and a new way of thinking are being established. We even saw increases in gamma activity overall, which meant improvement in the ability to make connections between memories in disparate parts of the brain and process information in an integrated and wise way.

> New thoughts are formed over twenty-one days, and these new thoughts are formed into habits after sixty-three days.

We saw these new thoughts become automatized (established as a habit) over the next forty-two days. By day 63, the experimental group had literally *transformed* their minds and the structure of their brains (neuroplasticity), sustaining this new way of thinking. This highlights something many of us intrinsically understand: it takes time to learn and form new habits that will impact how we function.

New thoughts are formed over twenty-one days, and these new thoughts are formed into habits after sixty-three days. This is extremely important to learning and life, because there are a lot of myths surrounding habit formation happening over just twenty-one days. This myth seems to have been started by a self-help book written by a cosmetic surgeon in 1960, and has been repeated so often that it's become an entrenched concept, but it's not factual.[3] My clinical trial adds additional evidence to a 2010 UK study on habit formation, and both indicate that habits form over at *least* sixty-three days, and some may take even longer—they need time to become automatized as useful information that will impact behavior in both the short and long term.[4]

Unmanaged Toxic Stress Impacts Our Brain and Blood

Throughout this trial, we also looked at the impact of mind-management techniques using the 5 Steps on mental and physical well-being in various blood measures such as homocysteine, cortisol, DHEA, ACTH, and prolactin, which are influenced by our lifestyle choices. We were curious to see if the dramatic changes we were seeing in the brain, the psychosocial data, and at the cellular level at day 21 and day 63 were also evident in the bloodwork.

Often, changes in the blood lag behind changes we see in the brain and in the mind, which is not surprising since the conscious mind lags behind the nonconscious mind by at least ten seconds.[5] We actually see changes in the qEEG *before conscious awareness of what's going on*. We were curious at what point we would find changes in the bloodwork of the experimental group. Initially, when we reviewed the data, it seemed that the blood results were all over the place. We were not completely surprised at this finding, because changes in bloodwork are often considered a secondary outcome, not the primary outcome, when looking at mental health.

However, what we did pick up when comparing bloodwork results with the results of the LMM scale was a *significant* relationship between unmanaged toxic stress and elevated levels of cortisol and homocysteine in the blood. This finding is notable, because it underscores the impact of unmanaged toxic stress on our physical health (the mind-brain-body connection). Unmanaged toxic stress is correlated with elevated cortisol and homocysteine levels, which puts people at risk for health issues like

> As the subjects managed their toxic stress using the 5 Steps of mind-management, they improved their homocysteine and cortisol levels significantly.

cardiovascular problems, immune system disorders, and neurological issues, including the dementias.

But there is good news! In our trial, as the subjects managed their toxic stress using the Neurocycle, *they improved their homocysteine and cortisol levels significantly*. So, not only did the experimental group significantly reduce their risk of mental health issues but they also potentially reduced their risk for cardiovascular concerns and other health issues. This is a very important finding!

The More the Mental Mess We Have, the Greater the Impact on Our DNA

On a cellular level, we also observed several fascinating changes. Telomere length (TL) has recently emerged as a proxy measure of biological aging and a correlate of severe stress, which means that the more unmanaged toxic stress you have in your life, the more your telomeres will shorten, and this is bad for your mental and physical health. A telomere is a structure at the end of a chromosome, a bit like the plastic at the end of a shoelace. It's very important for cell health because when it wears out and "frays," the cell will age more quickly and won't be as effective in keeping us healthy— much like a shoelace becomes hard to thread when it frays. Each time cells divide, they rely on telomeres, among many other factors, to do this properly, so the goal is to keep a healthy TL.

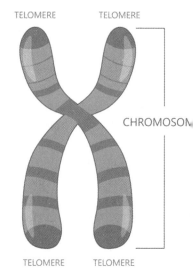

As we looked at telomere length and percentiles in our clinical trial over a nine-week period, the experimental group showed an

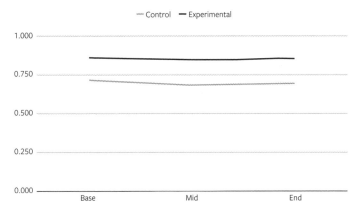

The difference in change of telomere length between the control group and experimental group over the course of the study. The experimental group, who had a mind-management strategy and therefore were able to manage their toxic stress, maintained a stable telomere length throughout the study. The control group, on the other hand, who were not given a mind-management strategy, showed a decrease in telomere length over sixty-three days—a change that it often takes years to see. Rapid decreases in telomere length have been associated with premature aging.

increased trend in length and the control group showed a decreased trend in length. There are emerging studies indicating that changes in TL can happen over short periods of time, and that interventions that target deliberate and intentional mind work (like the 5 Steps) can increase TL and potentially improve cellular health.[6]

Our study also assessed the association between telomere length and the implementation of mind-management techniques, specifically the Neurocycle. Over the course of the study, the experimental group's TL increased as they used the 5 Steps of the Neurocycle process, while the control group, who had no clear mind-management strategy, saw a decrease in TL. This is so important because telomeres have a lot to do with cellular health; the shorter your telomeres are, the unhealthier you will be, mentally and physically, and your vulnerability to disease will increase dramatically.

This clinical trial adds to the body of research showing that managing toxic stress is critical to our health. Telomere length varies widely between adults, and these findings suggest that mind-management could explain some of these differences. The deliberate, intentional, self-regulated thinking associated with the 5-Step process appears to promote a healthy biochemical milieu, which, in turn, could improve cell longevity.

We observed a similar pattern regarding the subjects' telomeres and relative age percentile. The control group's relative age percentile decreased over the course of the study, which means that they got biologically older, whereas the experimental group's percentiles held stable—*their biological age stayed the same.* This means that if we don't manage our minds, the organs in our physical bodies will get older than our actual chronological age. For example, we had one subject at the beginning of the study whose biological age was nearly twenty years older than actual chronological age—they were in their midthirties but had a body age of a fifty-year-old.

There's a significant amount of research indicating that the suppression of thoughts, which causes mental distress, is related to telomere shortening and biological aging. Suppressing thoughts can lead to psychological inflexibility—a sort of pretending to oneself that the thoughts don't exist. This suppression, in turn, affects cell health, which means organ health. Suppressing thoughts affects our heart, brain, GI system, and so on.

In our study, we observed that the subjects who did not want to deal with their suppressed thoughts and feelings also had more negative qEEG and telomere results. Changes indicated increased high beta and delta when correlated with measures that assessed thought suppression. This is unsurprising, as other research has shown that high beta activity is associated with anxiety; lots of high delta during the day generally indicates suppressed toxic thoughts, which results in factors such as poor sleep quality.

Life Experiences Are Reflected in Our Biology

What does all this data mean? When the body and brain are in a highly tense state, seen as multiple areas of high beta and low alpha activity on our qEEG results, as well as erratic changes in bloodwork and shortened TL, it can cause cellular aging, which impacts our physical health and our mental well-being over the short and long term. A restless mind can also leave the body in a chronically stressed-out state, and this unmanaged toxic stress suppresses the ongoing housekeeping and restorative functions of cell repair and puts the body into a low-grade state of inflammation, which can also accelerate the aging process.

The bottom line is that our *life experiences are reflected in our biology*, including our TL. However, mind-management interventions, like the Neurocycle tool used in our clinical trial, appear to act as a reset that enables us to restore our system to a healthier, younger state characterized by longer telomeres; more balanced energy flow of delta, theta, alpha, beta, and gamma; and significantly reduced homocysteine and cortisol levels, as well as an improved DHEA/cortisol ratio. As the subjects practiced using the 5 Steps, they had more balanced brain function and neuroplasticity and felt better and more empowered.

The LMM scale was able to pick up on this mindset shift, since it was more sensitive to the changes happening on the nonconscious level. We also observed these changes in the qEEG results more than in other clinical scales such as the Hospital Anxiety and Depression Scale (HADS) and Patient Health Questionnaire (PHQ). These more traditional scales, which are questionnaires used in hospital and mental health settings, tended to pick up only how the subject was feeling in the *now* moment. This is perhaps because the questions are very direct and leading. For example, the identity of self is reflected in the frontal cortex of the brain, and when we examined the qEEG data, that area didn't change very much over the period of the study in either the experimental or the control group. This suggests that the subjects were still *identifying with the label* of being depressed or anxious, so when asked a question in a leading way, as on the HADS and PHQ, they answered in a certain way because they still thought of themselves as a "depressed" person. They had not made the transition yet on a conscious level to being a person who is not depressed or anxious, even though they were not experiencing symptoms of depression and anxiety.

They did, however, show improvement in the LMM, qEEG, and narrative measures, which represent the nonconscious level of thinking—that is, where the deep level of processing occurs and where what you're *really* thinking and believing about yourself reside. This incongruence undergirds the dangers of labeling people with a mental illness. Such labeling appears to affect their perceived identity, potentially keeping them stuck in a certain mode of thinking even as they are going through the process of healing.

> Labeling people with a mental illness can affect their perceived identity and possibly remove their autonomy, instilling a sense of helplessness.

Why is this so important? A person who continues to identify with being depressed or anxious may choose to give up on therapy or a mind-management strategy because they're not aware they are improving, even though there's evidence in their nonconscious mind that they are getting better. The label seems to remove their autonomy and instill a sense of helplessness. They're not empowered to continue the hard work required during the healing process.

On the other hand, knowing that changes are occurring beneath the surface, on a nonconscious level, can be a powerful motivator, because it brings with it a sense of autonomy, encouraging someone to persist with therapy and mind-management techniques even if they don't feel different for some time. This is similar to when you're first trying to become fitter or lose weight, and you don't immediately see or feel different but you're empowered to keep going because you're aware of how your muscles are developing and how fat is being lost on the inside before it's evident on the outside. In fact, when it comes to exercise, your nervous system changes first, followed by your muscles.

> True change takes time and effort—there is no escaping this, no magic pill when it comes to our thinking.

True change takes time and effort—there's no escaping it, no magic pill when it comes to our thinking. Working on something like identifying toxic issues needs to be approached not as a one-off 63-day event but rather as an ongoing lifestyle. We're always going to be fixing something in our mental space, so this is a lifetime commitment. Knowing scientifically that it takes sixty-three days (a defined period of time) is empowering, because as humans we love defined periods; they reduce uncertainty in what may otherwise be a very uncertain process.

Using mind-management techniques such as the Neurocycle method will help you form an *ongoing delivery system* to keep your mind in that mental space where you're always managing what you're thinking, feeling, and choosing.

> *Both my son and I are doing the 5-Step program. He has high functioning autism. He worked on the fear of making mistakes and was engaged the entire way and worked hard to process. At day 21 he was excited and danced with big smiles on his face. I've never seen him feel so accomplished and happy about something this meaningful. He is gaining clarity, and he is less reactive against himself already after twenty-one days.*
>
> Kimberly

Chapter 4

The Research

Overview

- Your toxic stress and anxiety can be reduced by as much as 81 percent using the 5 Steps of the Neurocycle.

- Increased autonomy leads to increased awareness (because you learn to rely less on someone being aware for you, which is not always realistic or possible), or the sense that you can now self-regulate your toxic thoughts and reconceptualize them, which means your toxic stress levels will go down.

- As you use the 5 Steps daily, barriers and challenges that inevitably arise in life won't throw you as much—you will start seeing them as opportunities and possibilities!

- The 5 Steps can improve your overall psychological feelings of well-being, giving you a more positive outlook on life.

This is probably the most challenging chapter to get through, but it's so necessary because it undergirds the scientific nature of the Neurocycle method for mind-management. I want you to understand, experience, and know that as you are using this process, amazing and wonderful changes are happening in your brain and body even if you cannot immediately feel or see them, which is why I have included this rather technical chapter.

I also believe and know that challenging our minds to read difficult material is powerful and not only increases intelligence but also builds mental resilience—so just reading this chapter will make you smarter and mentally healthier! If you want more of the science, I invite you to read our white paper and the first of a series of journal publications in press.[1]

What follows is a summary of the study, highlighting the measures used and the overall results of our clinical trial. I have arranged the information to begin with an explanation of the *measure*, such as the Leaf Mind-Management Scale (LMM). Second are the results for the *control group*, who didn't have the Neurocycle app in the study. Third are the results of the *experimental group*, who did use the app, which took them through the 5 Steps for mind-management—they used this app daily as a guide through the process. And finally, each section concludes with an answer to the question, How does this help you? I have also included some graphs and qEEG head maps with explanations to help you visualize these results and the impact the mind-management process of the Neurocycle has on the brain (see color insert as well). Ready? Let's dig in.

Outline of Research

1. Psychosocial measures
2. Leaf Mind-Management Scale (LMM)
   a) Category 1: Autonomy
   b) Category 2: Awareness
   c) Category 3: Toxic thoughts
   d) Category 4: Toxic stress and anxiety

e) Category 5: Barriers and challenges

f) Category 6: Empowerment and life satisfaction

3. BBC Well-Being Scale

    a) Psychological

    b) Physical

    c) Relationships

4. Hospital Anxiety and Depression Scale (HADS)

    a) Anxiety

    b) Depression

5. Patient Health Questionnaire (PHQ)

    a) Depression

6. Narratives

7. Neurophysiological-electrical activity in the brain

    a) Frontal alpha asymmetry

    b) Frontal beta asymmetry

    c) Frontal gamma asymmetry

8. Physiology: bloodwork

    a) Homocysteine and cortisol

9. Cellular level: telomeres

1. Psychosocial Measures

Control Group

The control group showed an increased awareness of their is-sues, but the general trend across all measures was negative, sug-gesting that they became more aware but didn't have a way of managing them, so their self-regulation got worse over the course of the study.

Experimental Group

The experimental group showed an increase in awareness *and* self-regulation. There were positive changes in the psychosocial profiles in this group. The LMM was the most sensitive to these changes, which correlated with the qEEG. This reflects the work being done by the subjects; that is, what changes are happening on the nonconscious level.

2. Leaf Mind-Management Scale (LMM)

The LMM gives insight into what the subjects were really thinking on the nonconscious level over time. All LMM categories have dips at day 14, which correlated with changes in qEEG head maps at days 14 and 21. This is likely because from days 1 to 7, the subjects were beginning to increase in awareness (it can be quite shocking to see the mess in your mind!), while by day 14 things may have started coming together to the extent that subjects could get a little overconfident, thinking *I have improved; I have got this and can move on to the next thing that is worrying me!*

Category 1: Autonomy

Control Group

The control group did not have an upward trend in autonomy or feelings of control.

Experimental Group

Autonomy showed an upward trend in the experimental group. There is a marked difference between the experimental and control group in self-regulated autonomy.

How Does This Help You?

Autonomy is vital in terms of good self-regulation. It is linked to feelings of control, which means that subjects in the experimental group were sensing their own abilities: they could cope better with uncertainty, and they didn't always have to be reliant on therapists or coaches but could see them rather as facilitators and supporters. As our ability to manage our mind improves, our autonomy increases, which leads to feelings like *I've got this* or *I can handle this*. There is much research on how feelings of being in control of life and emotions can improve self-regulation and actual mental and physical health.[2] And the good news is that the more you use the Neurocycle, the more you will feel empowered and independent. We saw this in our research study: at the six-month mark, the experimental group was doing even better with their self-regulated mind-management skills than before. They got better and better over time with regular use of the Neurocycle! These same findings have been reported by thousands who have learned the 5 Steps from my books and app.

Category 2: Awareness

Control Group

The control group's increased awareness actually increased their anxiety, and they appeared to suppress their thoughts, which was seen in patterns in their brain. This seems to indicate a lack of insight into their issues, or even the choice not to face the issues, which led to burying the toxic thoughts. This was reflected in their qEEG results, which showed anxiety, depression, and toxic stress at different levels in all control group subjects.

Experimental Group

Awareness went from good to excellent in the experimental group. The experimental group refined their awareness, becoming more insightful, which enabled them to process through the situation they were working on. Their self-regulation was improving.

How Does This Help You?

This is exciting, as the 5 Steps focus on developing self-regulated awareness approximately every ten seconds, according to research, which simply means you can become increasingly sharp and self-aware, controlling your reactions and capturing thoughts when you are awake (conscious). Neuroscientific research indicates that we can change only what we are consciously aware of, because conscious awareness weakens the thought structures in the brain, making them more malleable to change. Even though facing things can be painful, it's comforting to know that doing so makes the thought structurally and emotionally weak.

With the combination of increased autonomy (category 1) and increased awareness, it becomes easier to deal with toxic thoughts,

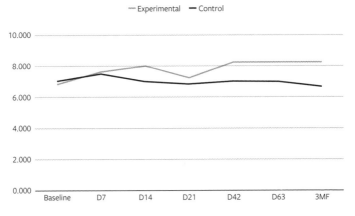

Changes in LMM subscale of awareness for both the experimental and control groups over the course of the study. The experimental group, shows an increase in awareness of the subjects' thoughts, emotions, and reactions over the course of the study, while the control group shows the opposite effect, a decrease in awareness throughout the time of the study.

and they will decrease over time because they are constantly being reconceptualized or reimagined. Essentially, the energy is being transferred from the toxic thoughts to healthy thoughts. Increased autonomy leads to the sense of *I can do this even though it's hard*, while increased awareness leads to the sense that *I can see what's going on, so now I can deal with my toxic thought* or *I can deal with the isolation, frustration, irritation, and so on.*

Category 3: Toxic Thoughts

Control Group

The control group's toxic thoughts generally got worse over time, as identified from their narrative and qEEG at each testing point of the study, especially by day 63, at which point the unmanaged toxic thoughts that had surfaced over the course of the study and had been pushed back down into the nonconscious mind were even more toxic than before.

Experimental Group

For the experimental group, toxic thoughts reduced significantly by day 14, and even more by day 63, and had really reduced by the six-month mark, showing a long-term effect of the Neurocycle and demonstrating the benefits of directed neuroplasticity.

How Does This Help You?

Toxic thoughts can be related to anything, from trauma to bad habits. As you learn the 5 Steps, your self-regulation will improve, and you will learn how to get these thought patterns under control, which can help increase your sense of empowerment and overall well-being. Part 2 of this book gives you the "know-how," including some 5-Step life hacks to get you through the day and on a pathway to self-regulated empowerment, just like the experimental group in our clinical trial!

Category 4: Toxic Stress and Anxiety

Control Group

The control group had increased toxic stress and anxiety the more aware they became of their negative thoughts. However, they didn't have any new tools to manage these thoughts, so they got worse.

Experimental Group

The experimental group showed the opposite effect: toxic stress and anxiety reduced significantly over the course of the study as they used the app and showed a sustainability effect at the six-month mark. So, they were increasingly aware of their toxic thoughts *and* their ability to manage them, indicated by their marked improvement (up to 81 percent!).

How Does This Help You?

Your toxic stress and anxiety can be reduced by as much as 81 percent using the Neurocycle; yes, you can learn how to do this! In fact, as you go through the 5 Steps, you are doing your own "brain surgery." Through this self-regulation, you are changing the interior design of your brain with mind-management.

Category 5: Barriers and Challenges

Control Group

Managing barriers and challenges worsened over the course of the study in the control group.

Experimental Group

Being able to manage and deal with the barriers and challenges of life improved for the experimental group, especially at the six-month mark of the study.

How Does This Help You?

As you use the Neurocycle daily, barriers and challenges that inevitably arise in life won't throw you as much—you will start seeing them as opportunities and possibilities, and you will get better and better at this as your self-regulation improves. This also implies that mind-management is a skill you can learn.

Category 6: Empowerment and Life Satisfaction

Control Group

The control group felt less empowered and less satisfied with life over the course of the study. This is possibly due to the fact that their increased awareness of their toxic mindsets also increased their toxic stress, while not having a specific mind-management strategy to deal with what they were becoming aware of made their issues worse.

Experimental Group

The experimental group showed an upward trend of empowerment and life satisfaction, which continued to improve across the study. This was reflected in the brain, as seen in the qEEG results.

How Does This Help You?

Increased autonomy will lead to increased awareness (because you learn to rely less on someone being aware for you, which is not always realistic or possible), the sense that you can now self-regulate your toxic thoughts and reconceptualize them, which means your toxic stress level will go down. You can then start to work on changing your perspective about how you are looking at the world. As you do this, you will start to see the situations of life as opportunities instead of negative challenges and barriers, all of which will increase your sense of empowerment and life satisfaction.

3. BBC Well-Being Scale

This scale is designed to measure a person's overall sense of "well-being" rather than studying specific measures of depression or anxiety. The BBC is divided into three sections and evaluates a person's overall psychological well-being, their physical well-being, and their relationships.

Psychological
Control Group

There was no measured improvement in the control group's well-being.

Experimental Group

There was significant measured improvement in the psychological well-being of the experimental group.

How Does This Help You?

The 5 Steps can improve your overall psychological feelings of well-being, giving you a more positive outlook on life.

Physical
Control Group

There was no improvement in the physical well-being of the control group.

Experimental Group

There was significant improvement in the physical well-being of the experimental group.

How Does This Help You?

The Neurocycle can improve your overall physical feelings of well-being, causing you to feel more energetic and ready for action.

Relationships

Control Group

There was no change in the well-being of relationships in the control group.

Experimental Group

There was a slight improvement in the well-being of relationships in the experimental group.

How Does This Help You?

The 5 Steps can improve your overall feelings of well-being in your relationships, helping you have more positive interactions with others.

4. Hospital Anxiety and Depression Scale (HADS)

The HADS is a screening test designed to measure a person's level of anxiety and depression over a short period of time. This is a self-assessment scale validated for use in both hospital and outpatient settings.

Anxiety

Control Group

The anxiety levels of the control group stayed the same throughout the study and showed no improvement.

Experimental Group

The experimental group reported statistically less anxiety compared to their baseline, even as far out as day 63. This was corroborated by the LMM and the qEEG and the themes highlighted in the narrative reports.

How Does This Help You?

When you use the 5 Steps, your self-regulation improves and you can start getting a handle on managing your anxiety. This doesn't mean it will go away entirely; you actually don't want it to, because anxiety is telling you something about your life that you need to know. It does mean, however, that your anxiety will decrease over time, and you will learn to manage it—it will work for you and not against you. Anxiety is not an illness; it is a warning signal that something needs attention in your life. It is normal to feel periods of anxiety. The Neurocycle method can help you find and manage what needs attention.

Depression

Control Group

There was no change in depression in the control group.

Experimental Group

At six months, the experimental group had statistically significantly less depression than the control group. This was corroborated by the LMM and the qEEG and the themes of the narrative.

How Does This Help You?

Using the 5 Steps can help you manage your depression. As with anxiety, depression is not an illness; it is a warning signal that something needs attention. The 5 steps can help you find this and process and reconceptualize it—and improve your mind and brain health as you do so.

5. Patient Health Questionnaire (PHQ)

The PHQ is not a screening test but instead is used to assess the severity of depression in a person and their response to treatment.

Depression

Control Group

There was no improvement in depression in the control group.

Experimental Group

The experimental group showed a significant treatment effect at days 1 to 7 and days 7 to 14. The treatment effect went away if subjects stopped using the 5 Steps and therefore stopped self-regulating.

How Does This Help You?

As we saw with the HADS, if you use the Neurocycle method consistently, you can deal with your depression in a meaningful and sustainable way, and you can start seeing this in your life as early as after one week of doing the 5 Steps daily.

6. Narratives

Narrative is the subjects' individual stories—their life and context. The experimental group subjects were asked to write out responses to a number of different open-ended questions that allowed us to analyze a total of sixteen different themes. We measured and statistically analyzed the number of times each of these themes was mentioned in the narratives at day 1, day 21, day 63, and at the six-month follow-up.

These themes were acceptance of challenges, anxiety, cancer, death and dying, decision-making, family, friends, job satisfaction, perspective taking, positive self-perceptions, sleep problems, suicide, support systems, traumatic experiences, unemployment, and work.

Experimental Group

The overall trend for the experimental group was an improvement in the majority of the narrative themes. So, for positive themes, such as acceptance of challenges, we gradually saw more instances mentioned in the narratives. And for negative themes, such as death and dying, we saw fewer instances as the study progressed. These improvements matched and were corroborated by LMM scores. Narratives and self-reporting indicated that although subjects were still battling some issues, they were able to deal with them more effectively, which demonstrates improvement in their self-regulation. Their reduction in anxious thoughts was the most dramatic at 81 percent; their decision-making, management of toxic thoughts, and management of barriers and challenges all showed marked improvement, and 25 percent reported improved sleep.

How Does This Help You?

Your narrative is your unique story that deserves to be heard; no one is an expert on your experience except you . . . you are your own case study! When people learn how to tell their own story, their lives change in ways they never imagined. When you feel you can control your own mind and life, you can live in peace and find healing regardless of your past, present, or future; we observed this in my clinical trials. Autonomy and independence are predictive of healing, while people who feel like everything is out of their control tend to be more susceptible to the fluctuations of life.

The 5 Steps can help you embrace, process, and reconceptualize this story. If your narrative stays inside of you—that is, if you suppress how you are feeling—this can damage your mind, brain, and body, which we observed in our study. However, because of the neuroplasticity of the brain, you can direct this change—you don't have to stay stuck in one way of thinking.

7. Neurophysiological-Electrical Activity in the Brain

Control Group

Changes observed in the control group indicated erratic brain activity at the nonconscious level, with negative changes in the electrical activity and neuroplasticity of the brain causing imbalance and decoherence, which damage brain and mind health.

Experimental Group

For the experimental group, changes observed in the qEEG indicated improved balance and coherence of the electrical activity in the brain, which correlated with psychosocial scales and narrative changes. This indicates that the process of conscious, intentional, directed neuroplasticity through mind-management had significant impact on the nonconscious level—that is, the process of embracing and processing to find the root issue and reconceptualize the new habit.

Frontal Alpha Asymmetry (FAA) Z Score

Frontal alpha asymmetry (FAA) measures the difference in electrical activity in the alpha frequency between the two halves of the brain. FAA is associated with depression, sadness, flatness in emotions, and identity issues. The brain likes coherence and balance, and we want to see a move to the midline on the graphs to show this. The more asymmetry (imbalance) between the left and right hemispheres of the frontal lobes, the more depression and mental mess we experience.

Control Group

No significant improvement took place in the control group. Very little or no flipping between hemispheres occurred, showing very little processing was happening. In fact, the asymmetry stayed the same or got worse.

Experimental Group

The experimental group showed an improved pattern in the balance between the two sides of the brain. They had more communication between the hemispheres as thoughts were being embraced, processed, and reconceptualized at day 21, which settled close to the midline around day 63. We saw this pattern happening in the front of the brain, which went from significant alpha asymmetry in the left hemisphere, which is associated with the warning signals of depression and sadness, to flipping sides to significant asymmetry in the right hemisphere by day 21, as facing the issues and finding the root of the depression took place. This significant alpha asymmetry at day 21 shows long-term memory was being built and there were a lot of feelings associated with this process, but by day 63 there was very little asymmetry between the two hemispheres, which is good, as it indicates coherence and a balanced brain. It also shows the significance of habit formation taking at least sixty-three days. Such flipping indicates processing is going on——that is, flipping between detail to big-picture processing on the left, and big-picture to detail processing on the right, which is what we want to see, as it indicates people are thinking deeply about their issues and not suppressing them. Those subjects who suppressed their thoughts or didn't manage them did not show this type of deep processing.

How Does This Help You?

Using the Neurocycle increases your self-regulation through mind-management. This changes the way energy in the brain flows as well as the structure of the brain when it comes to depression. This kind of directed neuroplasticity means you are changing your physical brain structure.

The energy flattens in a depressed brain; this is toxic to brain cells that need healthy energy flow to function. However, energy increases when we shift perception from seeing depression as an illness to seeing it as a warning signal with an underlying cause that can be identified and changed. Embracing, processing, and

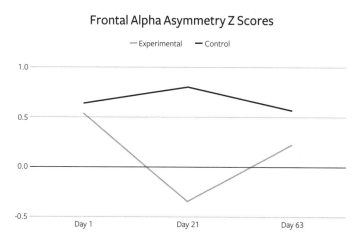

Frontal Alpha Asymmetry Z Scores

— Experimental   — Control

Changes in frontal alpha asymmetry for both the experimental and control groups over the course of the study. Negative numbers represent more alpha activity on the right side of the brain, suggesting subjects are focusing on the big picture to detail, while positive numbers represent more alpha activity on the left side of the brain, suggesting subjects are focusing on detail to the big picture. A "z score" of 0 indicates the balance of activity in an average person's brain, based on a large database of subjects. As you can see, both the experimental and control group started with activity more predominantly on the left side of the brain. The experimental group changed their way of thinking at day 21 to more of a big picture to detail thinking, and then by day 63, the electrical activity was closer to that of an "average" person without depression. In contrast, there is very little change in the alpha activity of the control group, which shows overthinking and/or ruminating.

reconceptualizing to find the source or root of depression can help change energy flow in the brain. You can literally heal your brain with your mind!

Frontal Beta Asymmetry

Frontal beta asymmetry measures the difference in electrical activity in the beta frequency between the two halves of the brain. Excessive high beta activity is associated with anxiety and identity problems. As with alpha activity, the brain likes coherence and balance, and we want to see a move to the midline on the graphs, which means the high beta activity reduces. The more asymmetry (imbalance) between the hemispheres, the more anxiety, identity issues, and mental mess.

Control Group

The control group did not show any marked improvement; in fact, their results indicated that their thinking was getting worse as they became more aware of their issues by taking the psychosocial and other measurement scales. High beta increased as their anxiety increased. There was a continual increased number of high beta foci (points) over the course of the study, especially across the midline, which reflected ruminating and not having cognitive flexibility as beta and gamma increased across the whole brain. So, awareness without a sustainable mind-management plan made them worse and not better.

Experimental Group

Subjects in the experimental group showed exciting and notable improvement, indicating their brains were becoming more balanced after embracing, processing, and reconceptualizing in response to using the 5 Steps of the Neurocycle method. This was seen initially as too much high beta, as described for the experimental group and which is what I call a "red brain." The subjects got a little more anxious on day 21 as they faced issues and built new thoughts, which is challenging, is hard, and can increase anxiety—things generally get worse before they get better. This was reflected in the brain as multiple foci of high bursts of beta, which is good because it indicated that the subjects were facing, not suppressing, their issues. By day 63 the subjects' qEEG results indicated habit formation. Their high beta became more cyclic and balanced across the left and right frontal lobes.

This is where we observed a huge difference between the experimental and control groups. The control group's high beta and gamma kept increasing "tsunami style," whereas the experimental group, with their mind-management skills gained from using the Neurocycle app, had cyclical increases and decreases, then balance. This indicates that they were gaining control and an increased ability to focus, pay attention, and think with more clarity.

How Does This Help You?

When you use the 5 Steps, you can change the way energy in your brain flows, from too much high beta activity on one side of the front part of the brain to cyclic high beta on both sides of the brain that is more balanced. In effect, you are "fixing" the damage from anxious thinking—you are regenerating your brain! When the energy is too high for too long, it affects your brain cells, which need healthy energy to function. For example, you can get stuck ruminating on an intrusive thought or a negative pattern, which can be seen as multiple red foci on the top of the brain over an area called the *corpus callosum*. This can lead to OCD-type behaviors or inflexibility and resistance to change in order to compensate. Embracing, processing, and reconceptualizing to find the source or root of the anxiety, depression, burnout, or patterns of thinking that are stuck, on the other hand, results in positive brain changes. The experimental group was getting "unstuck," turning their ruminating into progressive, problem-solving-type thinking as they used the 5 Steps.

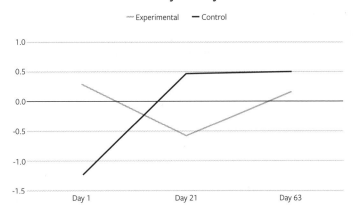

Frontal Beta Asymmetry Z Scores

Changes in frontal beta asymmetry for both the experimental and control groups over the course of the study. Negative numbers represent more beta activity on the right side of the brain, suggesting subjects are focusing on the big picture to detail, while positive numbers represent more beta activity on the left side of the brain, suggesting subjects are focusing on detail to the big picture. A "z score" of 0 indicates the balance of activity in an average person's brain, based on a large database of subjects. Interestingly, the experimental and control groups started with beta activity on different sides of the brain—the experimental group with more left-brain beta activity and the control group with more right-brain beta activity. The experimental group changed their way of thinking at day 21 to more of a big picture to detail thinking, then by day 63, the electrical activity was closer to that of an "average" person without anxiety, or a balance between big picture to detail and detail to big picture. The control group, although they did change from more right-sided beta activity to left-sided activity at day 21, did not show a trend closer to the qEEG patterns of an "average" person's brain; rather, they shifted how they were getting stuck in the detail, as indicated by the flat line.

Frontal Gamma Asymmetry

Frontal gamma asymmetry measures the difference in electrical activity in the gamma frequency between the two halves of the brain. Gamma activity is associated with learning, integrative thinking, and high level executive functioning and creativity. When we see gamma activity flipping sides and "gamma peaks," this means processing and learning are taking place in an organized fashion and neuroplasticity is being driven in the right direction.

We consider this to represent directed neuroplasticity. When we see gamma activity return to the right hemisphere, this means automatization (habit formation) is taking place.

Control Group

Data from the control group indicated they got stuck, with minimal learning taking place at day 21. Thoughts were being drawn into conscious awareness but were going back into the nonconscious mind (being suppressed) because they weren't managed, so they were in fact going back worse than before, increasing their negative impact. The results indicate that in the control group very little learning took place; the peak where real learning takes place and reconceptualization happens didn't occur in the control group, and instead we observed a flattened peak. There was also increased anxiety. When undealt-with thoughts are suppressed, they become stronger than they were before, affecting anxiety levels and mental health.

Experimental Group

Data from the experimental group shows learning taking place with the gamma activity increasing at day 21, forming "gamma peaks," and the return of gamma activity closer to baseline at day 63, which suggests that the thoughts were being automatized into habits. Interestingly, we saw these gamma "peaks" only in the experimental subjects who *completed* sixty-three days using the app, which indicates a lot of learning took place. Some of the experimental subjects stopped using the app after one or two 21-day cycles, and we saw changes in gamma in those subjects more in line with the control group.

How Does This Help You?

When you use the Neurocycle for mind-management, you are learning how to direct your neuroplasticity to grow the kind of thoughts in your brain that will help you feel empowered and improve your well-being. As you think deeply and build new thoughts (learning), you will experience an improvement in brain function; you will actually be changing the structure of your brain in a positive direction. This is the hard work of digging into your nonconscious mind and getting comfortable with the uncomfortable; for example, you may start seeing your breakdowns as good because you can use them to reconceptualize your toxic thoughts and trauma. You yourself are not breaking down; rather, you are empowered by *doing* the "breaking down"—such breakdowns mean façades being pulled down!

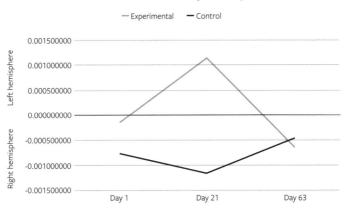

Changes in frontal gamma asymmetry for one subject in the experimental group who used the SWITCH app throughout the entire clinical trial and a subject from the control group. Negative numbers represent more gamma activity on the right side of the brain, suggesting subjects are focusing on the big picture to detail, while the positive numbers represent more gamma activity on the left side of the brain, suggesting subjects are focusing on detail to the big picture. There are no "z scores" for gamma activity, as this was not a frequency that was studied at the time the z score database was created. So, the values you see here are millivolts of gamma activity. We see a clear "gamma peak" in the experimental subject, with increasing gamma activity at day 21, then decreasing gamma activity by day 63, suggesting that the learning phase had transitioned to a habit being formed. By contrast, the control subject showed very little change in gamma activity at any of the time points; they were not changing and, therefore, not "growing" through the experience.

8. Physiology: Bloodwork

Blood values have many potential variables and are therefore not reliable measures of anxiety and depression, which is why they should not be used to define a person's level of anxiety or depression. They are more of an indication of the resultant wear and tear of anxiety and depression on the body.

Control Group

The most notable bloodwork trends in the control group involved negative homocysteine and cortisol levels.

Experimental Group

We studied a number of blood measures in this clinical trial, including homocysteine, cortisol, prolactin, ACTH, and DHEA levels. The most notable positive trends in the experimental group involved their homocysteine and cortisol levels.

Homocysteine and Cortisol

Control Group

In the control group, the lack of mind-management led to an increase in homocysteine and cortisol levels.

Experimental Group

In the experimental group, there was a marked positive relationship between toxic stress and homocysteine and cortisol, indicating that individuals with higher toxic stress scores on the LMM had higher homocysteine and cortisol levels in their blood.

There was also a significant positive relationship between the change in toxic stress and the change in homocysteine, indicating that, as individuals used the 5 Steps over the course of the study, their toxic stress scores on the LMM lowered, and they also had lower homocysteine and cortisol levels in their blood. This also led to an improved DHEA/cortisol ratio, which is an indicator of how stress affects the hypothalamic-pituitary-adrenal (HPA) axis. So, if stress is unmanaged and toxic, the DHEA/cortisol ratio drops, and vice versa.

Comparatively, individuals with worse toxic stress scores on the LMM had higher homocysteine and cortisol in the blood. This supports the link between high stress, high homocysteine, and high cortisol, and suggests that reducing toxic stress through mind-management not only lowers homocysteine but may also help prevent cardiovascular concerns and autoimmune issues and potentially lower someone's risk for neurological issues.

How Does This Help You?

We found a notably significant relationship between unmanaged toxic stress and elevated cortisol and homocysteine levels and DHEA/cortisol ratios, which suggests that as you improve how you manage toxic stress using the 5 Steps, you can potentially improve your homocysteine and cortisol levels and DHEA/cortisol ratio, which not only reduces your risk of mental ill-health but may also reduce your risk for cardiovascular concerns, autoimmune issues, and neurological issues, including the dementias.

9. Cellular Level: Telomeres

Telomeres are the caps on the ends of chromosomes and are very important to cellular health and biological aging. Telomere length (TL) has recently emerged as a proxy measure of biological aging and correlates to severe stress. Shorter telomeres are a chromosome component associated with cellular aging and toxic stress, and TL is now on the map as one of the most consistent predictors of shorter life span!

Control Group

The TL of the control group decreased from baseline by the end of the study. This suggests that without mind-management, the control subjects' cellular health and biological age were negatively impacted.

Experimental Group

Using the Neurocycle method was correlated with increased TL in the experimental group, suggesting that the experimental subjects' cellular health and biological age improved over the course of the study.

How Does This Help You?

Using the 5 Steps can potentially increase your cellular health and improve your biological age, which means the health of your heart, brain, GI tract, immune system, and so on. Suppressing or trying to avoid unhappy toxic thoughts causes distress right down to the cellular level, which can shorten telomeres and potentially increase biological age in relation to chronological age (your body can age faster than your actual age) which increases vulnerability to physical illnesses.

You may think you are getting away with not dealing with your stuff, but your brain, body, and mind will eventually pay the price. Psychological inflexibility, attachment to maintaining a positive air, and the avoidance of negative situations may help you suppress unwanted thoughts or feelings in the present moment but will create fertile ground for more frequent or exaggerated breakdowns in the long term. Basically, gene activity (not gene sequences) changes in response to our life experiences and this activity can be beneficial or harmful depending on how we are thinking. When your thinking is toxic, things may seem worse than what they are, and it can be difficult to get perspective.

Avoidance can damage the cells of our body via aging our telomeres, which can impact our mental health. Our life experiences are reflected in telomere length. However, mind-management interventions like the 5 Steps of the Neurocycle used in this clinical trial might act as a "reset," inducing critical periods where we can "shake up" our system to develop a healthier, younger state.

I did multiple cycles of the 5-Step program and today I celebrate fifteen months completely off anxiety medication. I feel grateful, peaceful, empowered, and free!"

BONNIE

Chapter 5

How Can All This Science Help You?

Overview

- Even if we still feel anxious or depressed, acknowledging, embracing, and processing our issues will optimize brain function and create coherence, which will give us the ability to see our issues clearly and deal with them.

- Uncontrolled, toxic thinking has the potential to create a state of low-grade inflammation across the body and brain, adversely affecting cortisol levels, hormones, brain functionality, and even the telomeres on the chromosomes.

- People who have been taught to "tune in" to their nonconscious mind to manage their thought life and "detox" and "build" the brain are better able to navigate the ups and downs of life because they have a sense of control, which gives them hope.

Our clinical trial results, when viewed alongside the observed changes in the experimental group's scores on my validated Leaf Mind-Management Scale (LMM) are exciting. They demonstrate that subjects who used the 5 Steps in the Neurocycle app transitioned from awareness of their toxic thinking *without* a mind-management strategy to an ability to independently process and reconceptualize their toxic thoughts *with* the specific 5-Step mind-management technique. In short, they moved from awareness of having a problem to being empowered to work out how to deal with and overcome their problem.

So, this is what the science means for you: you can transition from just being aware of your chaotic and toxic thoughts to being empowered to catch these thoughts in their early stages, manage them, and improve your overall peace and well-being. With appropriate mind-management training and self-regulation, which is what "cleaning up the mental mess" using the Neurocycle is all about, we can systematically use our mind to take advantage of the neuroplasticity of our brain to rework and rewire our thoughts. In part 2 of this book I show you how to do this.

We can transform our neural circuitry, which enables us to manage and improve a variety of mental and physical states. This means we can literally take dysfunctional brain networks and physiology and alter them with our mind. We can manage our thinking and clean up the mental mess with habit-forming cycles of sixty-three days that give a new thought pattern enough energy to become a habit that influences our behavior and communication. And if this is done continually, as a lifestyle, overall well-being, peace, and wisdom are the reward.

As you learn to use the information and the Neurocycle provided in this book, you'll become equipped to prevent the development of toxic thoughts, reconceptualize traumatic thoughts, and change and improve all areas of your life, including managing depression, anxiety, and burnout that can come from chronic and recurrent stress, trauma, identity issues, isolation, sleep difficulties, challenges with exercise and diet, and so much more. The 5-Step process uses all the benefits of breathing and mindfulness, taking these into the realm of long-term, sustainable mind-management.

Yes, it will take time, it will be challenging, and it's a lifelong process, but you are always thinking anyway, so you may as well try to learn to manage the process—and the changes will be worth it. It was incredibly exciting to see that after twenty-one days of using the app, there was up to an 81 percent reduction in depression and anxiety in the experimental group versus the control group in our clinical trial.

This can be *your* story too.

qEEG and Brain Coherence

Using specific neuroscientific measures (qEEG), we found that as the subjects in the experimental group started managing their minds, the energy and functionality in their brains became more balanced and coherent, which optimized brain function and allowed their thinking to become more coherent. You can think of *coherence* as many parts of the brain working together in harmony. Our brains are always generating energy in response to how we think, feel, and choose, and the more we deal with our stuff, the more coherence we will see in our brain and the clearer we'll be able to think and the more resilient we'll become. When the energy in the brain drops too low in the frontal lobe and loses coherence between the two sides, it can result in depression and impulsivity and the feeling of just wanting to give up.

Even if we still feel anxious or depressed, acknowledging, embracing, and processing our issues will optimize brain function and create coherence, which will give us the ability to see our issues clearly and deal with them. On the other hand, if we suppress our problems and try to convince ourselves that we've dealt with them, or use techniques or positive affirmations as a Band-Aid rather than seeking a long-term solution, we will create *incoherence* in the brain, which, over time, can lead to a variety of mental and physical issues.

We observed this in our study. A qEEG (quantitative electro-encephalogram) is not reading a single thought—no brain technology can read your thoughts. You are not your brain; you are the "user" of your brain. The qEEG is picking up this energy *response* in the brain to what a person is thinking, feeling, and choosing in any one moment. It reflects the nonconscious mind energy levels, where our intelligence, memories (good and bad), and wisdom reside, including any *cognitive dissonance*, which is the discrepancy between what we truly feel and what we say we feel or are trying to convince ourselves to feel.

For example, let's say you live, act, and speak according to a restrictive religious, cultural, familial, or work environment. Perhaps there are some things you observe that don't sit well with you, or you feel like you're acting a role, doing and saying what's expected of you but not what you believe. At the back of your mind is a room where the truth is, but your fear won't let that truth out of the room. Eventually, you feel like you cannot live the lie anymore; you feel it in your body and in your mind. The lie is eating you alive: you feel like you've lost your integrity, your truth value. In the brain, this will look like incoherence or imbalance—messy energy, kind of like the rapids of whitewater rafting. We can't hide what we're thinking from our brains—the brain will reflect any anxiety, depression, and frustration. This is what a qEEG, SPECT, and other brain technology methods pick up, and this is the kind of mental mess we want to get rid of. (To see what this looks like in the brain, see the "Subject 2 qEEG Z Scores" image in the color insert.)

> What value do you give peace and freedom in your mind?

There will come a time when you simply have to make the choice as to whether you stay chained or get free, no matter what the cost. And the cost of integrity can be very high, but so are the rewards on the other side! Indeed, I would ask you: What value do you give peace and freedom in your mind?

It's in the quiet stillness of the moment, when we think deeply about our thinking, that we can draw on our courage to go into the depths of our nonconscious mind and embrace the chaos to find the message of truth.

Your mind loves this. Your brain loves this. You will love the peace this eventually brings.

Coherent and Incoherent Brain Waves

To better understand what I mean by coherence and incoherence, let's look at two EEG images from my clinical trial. The first is a subject in the experimental group who was going through some major stuff and had experienced significant early childhood trauma, but was using the 5-Step process to manage their issues. This EEG reading shows coherence and balance. For this person, this felt like peace and control and resilience despite the adverse experiences. They were learning to manage the feeling of being overwhelmed. The second image is from a subject in the control group and reflects what it looks like when someone does not manage their mind: it shows incoherence and what a mental mess looks like in the brain. For this person, this incoherence resulted in a hypervigilant stress state—they were in a perpetual switched "on" state of high anxiety, and had no peace.

An Experimental Subject's Story: Learning to Manage Depression

Let's take a look at one person's story from the experimental group to help you make sense of all the data.

Turn to the first page of the color insert to find "Subject 1 qEEG Z Scores," the qEEG head map of this person. At baseline (day 1

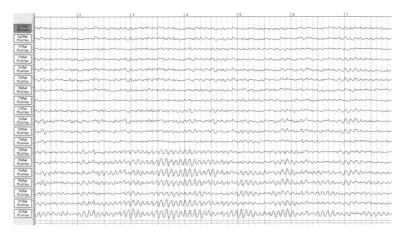

A snippet of an EEG recording from an experimental group subject, showing coherence across all areas of the brain. Note how patterns of waves of electrical activity appear to be fairly uniform across all electrodes, represented by rows.

A snippet of an EEG recording from a control group subject, showing incoherence of the electrical activity in the brain. The patterns of wave activity are very different in the different rows, representing differing levels of electrical activity in many of the electrodes, that reflect incoherence, or disharmony, in the brain.

of the clinical trial), the subject reported feeling significantly depressed; wasn't sleeping, was battling with memory and relationship issues at home and at work, and felt burned out, emotionally exhausted, unhappy, and cynical.

At day 1, the blue color indicates significantly lower than average energy in the brain across all frequencies. It is specifically low and unbalanced in the front of the brain. This pattern is consistent with a person who is severely depressed. By day 21, the energy in their brain has increased—as indicated by the gray color, which represents the average or expected brain activity in a nondepressed person, as compared to a normative database.

The experimental subject's qEEG pattern was still improving at day 63 as their mind-management skills using the Neurocycle method continued to improve. Neuropsychological measures and narrative data demonstrated that the improvement in symptoms of depression and anxiety in the subject was sustained at a follow-up at the six-month mark of the study, which was evident in their neuroscientific data and bloodwork.

Essentially, this means that the subject was increasing their self-regulation and *learning* to identify and deal with the cause of their depression. They were learning how to manage their thinking on a daily basis and as a lifestyle—they were

> The subject was learning to identify the cause of their depression and manage their mind over the course of sixty-three days.

using neurocycling to direct their neuroplasticity. This data was supported by their neuropsychological self-reporting scales and their narrative, which described that they no longer felt severely depressed and had less anxiety, burnout, cynicism, and emotional exhaustion. They were sleeping better and felt that they had the skills in place to cope. They also felt like they had increased mental resilience and felt more empowered to deal with the barriers and challenges they were facing in their life.

What is really interesting with this subject is that at day 1, they were quite insightful and aware of their issues and had tried everything to help deal with their depression. This insight is indicated by the flares of green in the alpha frequency, along with the flares of green in the frontal lobe in the delta frequency in the image above. However, the blues, particularly the darker blue colors, indicated that *they did not know what to do about how they felt—the deep sense of "everything is just too much."* This finding was corroborated by the subject's narrative description of their experience, which suggested they felt stuck, helpless, and hopeless, and by their psychosocial test scores, specifically the results on the LMM and narrative, as well as their telomere data (DNA health). Their cortisol and homocysteine levels were also problematic at the beginning of the study, indicating low-grade inflammation across their brain and body, which is one more indicator of poor brain health.

However, by day 21, this feeling of not knowing what to do had changed to a kind of actionable insight, a sense of empowerment. The subject felt they were starting to process and reconceptualize what was making them feel depressed and were developing the courage to face and embrace their thoughts, which made them feel both hopeful and ill at ease. They felt hopeful that they were starting to get insight into their issues, but ill at ease because it's painful to face and deal with problems. As they say, the night is darkest before dawn, and often things get worse before they get better. We could see this in the qEEG by the increased activity in the alpha frequency, indicated by the gray color.

How Does This Help You?

There's no straightforward, quick, magic solution when it comes to healing the mind and cleaning up our mental mess. When deep,

hidden wounds are exposed, there's always pain before healing—
both physically and mentally. It's important we prepare ourselves
for this so we don't get thrown when we feel we should be getting
better but actually feel worse at first. It's
a good idea to have a support system in
place: a trusted confidante, therapist, or
counselor to talk to in the tougher moments. And remember to give yourself
mental health breaks in the process.

> When deep, hidden wounds are exposed, there's always pain before healing—both physically and mentally.

It's also important to remind yourself
that "this too shall pass." As you persist
with mind-management, you're rewiring
your brain for the better, which can be
painful, but you will experience freedom
on the other side. You will learn to tol-
erate more emotional difficulty without
falling apart or feeling guilt or shame as you go through something.
This will help you feel more present with yourself and your loved
ones. There's no shame in this. In fact, the feelings you experience
are important—they are an awareness of your humanity.

Let's look back at the subject from the experimental group.
By day 63, they were self-regulating and managing their thoughts
around what had been making them depressed. We observed flares
of green at the beta frequency on the back left of the head map,
which indicated their brain was online and their conscious mind
was working with their nonconscious mind to create a new type
of expectancy that was helping them cope. In effect, they were
starting to believe things would get better because they started
seeing things get better.

Subject 1: Frontal Alpha Asymmetry and Beta Asymmetry Eyes Open

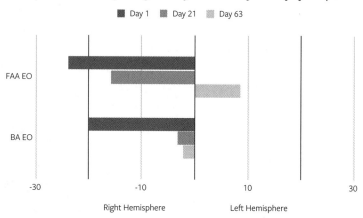

Changes in alpha and beta activity, based on qEEG data, over the course of study for this experimental subject. Alpha activity decreases at day 21 on the right side, indicating more balance in the alpha activity, which is associated with less depression. We see by day 63 that the alpha activity has now switched to the left side of the brain and is much more balanced than at the beginning of the study. Likewise, the beta activity significantly decreases at day 21 compared to baseline, indicating that this subject is experiencing much less anxiety. This effect is sustained at day 63.

Subject 1: Frontal Gamma Asymmetry Eyes Open

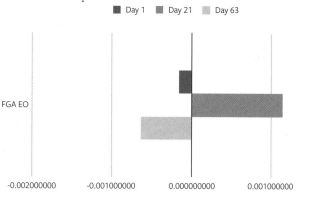

Changes in gamma activity, based on qEEG data, over the course of study for this experimental subject. Gamma activity increases and switches from the right hemisphere to the left hemisphere at day 21, indicating learning. This is a gamma "peak," which is a good thing because it's showing change happening in the subject's mind, and this change is being reflected in the subject's brain. By day 63, gamma activity has decreased and switched back to the right side of the brain, which is also a good thing because it suggests that this learning has turned into a habit and the subject's positive changes will be sustainable.

As we look at the line graph for gamma activity in this subject in the figure below, we also see a "gamma peak" that indicates learning is taking place, as mentioned above.

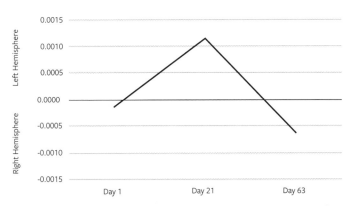

Subject 1: Gamma Frontal Asymmetry Eyes Open

Another way to look at gamma activity, based on qEEG data, over the course of study for the same experimental subject. We see gamma activity switch from the right hemisphere to the left hemisphere (negative values to positive values) and then return to the right hemisphere—forming a "gamma peak" associated with learning and then solidifying the learning to form a habit.

How Does This Help You?

When people get into toxic thinking habits, it can mess up the stress response. The stress response is actually good for us if it's part of a balanced lifestyle, just like exercise is a type of good stress on the body. Think about taking a test: a healthy stress response helps us stay energized, focused, and awake, which boosts our mental performance. However, if we start panicking in the middle of the test, we start experiencing mental fog and can't think clearly—that is toxic stress, and it occurs when we let our thoughts run amok.

Toxic stress is no joke. Psychoneuroimmunology research has shown how conscious thinking controls the function of the immune system—when we stress, we impact the body's ability to protect itself. In fact, research has shown how healthy and con-structive thinking can lead to the *placebo effect*, allowing the mind to fight disease, while toxic thinking can create the *nocebo effect*, which can increase our vulnerability to disease.

Toxic stress has been demonstrated as being responsible for up to 90 percent of illness, including heart disease, cancer, and diabetes.[1] When an individual is in a toxic thinking state, the release of stress hormones such as cortisol, ACTH, and even prolactin shut down the immune system to conserve the body's energy for the flight-or-fight response. This is good if you're running away from a threat, getting ready for the day, need to be focused in a business presentation, or dealing with a relational crisis. However, stress works in cycles of tension and release, and if the release does not come—if this state of stress response becomes chronic—we get in the habit of perceiving the physical sensations of stress as bad for us instead of good for us.[2] We then react negatively to daily stressors over long periods of time, which compromises instead of enhances the immune system.

> Using mind-management techniques like the 5 Steps of the Neurocycle, you can learn how to make your stress response work for you and not against you.

In this experimental subject, we saw this type of elevated cortisol and homocysteine at day 1, and then saw it reduce over the course of the study. As the subject learned how to manage their mind, the body's cortisol and homocysteine came back into balance, highlighting the integration be-tween the mind and the body. We also saw this subject's telomeres lengthen and the biological age decrease over the course of the six months of the clinical trial in response to their learning to make stress work for them and not against them.

So, as you learn how to manage your thinking using mind-management techniques like the 5 Steps presented in this book, *you* can learn how to make your stress response work for you and not against you. This, in turn, can boost both your mental and physical health, improving the communication between your mind and body.

A Control Subject's Story: from Anxiety to More Anxiety

Turn to the second page of the color insert to find "Subject 2 qEEG Z Scores," the qEEG head map of this person. This subject, a Millennial, was part of the control group, which means they weren't given the intervention (the 5-Step mind-management program via the SWITCH app). They did, however, complete the evaluation instruments, including our LMM scale, bloodwork, telomere evaluation, and qEEG studies at the different time points of the study.

During the course of our study, this subject reported feeling slammed and overwhelmed by life. Everything was too much: work, relationships, financial pressure, and so on. This was corroborated by their narrative and self-reported well-being scores, as well as the anxiety, depression, and self-regulation psychological evaluations they filled out seven times over the six months of the study. These evaluation instruments are designed to increase self-awareness of how subjects are feeling emotionally and how they're functioning mentally, including what kind of lifestyle decisions they're making and how these are impacting their day-to-day activities.

The subject's qEEG showed patterns that suggested they were suffering from extreme anxiety, experiencing frequent panic attacks, and not sleeping well because of the pressure they felt from everything in their life, which is not an uncommon story these days. They ruminated a lot, battled with intrusive thoughts, and felt very stuck. These feelings affected their brain energy and blood physiology.

At day 1, their brain had a lot of high beta activity over the amygdala region, an area that we use to respond to and process emotional perceptions—see the "red brain." This suggests they were highly anxious and distressed and reflects a pattern of intrusive thoughts and ruminating. The amygdala is like a perceptual library filled with books containing the emotional perceptions attached to our thoughts. Too much activity here is like reading too many books about the bad things that can happen and obsessively thinking about what you just read.

When we get into this state, we tend to overreact, overgeneralize, and even catastrophize situations. We can easily get into the kind of thinking patterns that overexaggerate yesterday's issues while overemphasizing tomorrow's and undervaluing the significance of what's happening today and how we can change things. The poor brain, which does the bidding of the mind, has all the wrong energy flow through the internal networks, and the memories, which are stored as energy vibrations in proteins on the branches of the neurons, cause them to experience earthquake-like shakes. Staying in this pattern means, unfortunately, that the earthquake can end up doing a lot of damage, which is what we observed happening with the subject in the clinical trial. However, with mind-management and support, we can get out of this type of negative spiral, which is why all the subjects in the control group were given access to the Neurocycle program when the study was over.

How Does This Help You?

We need to understand that our thinking is real and has real effects on the brain. If we don't manage our mind, we can fall into the trap of living in a "nether world" where everything feels terrible and hopeless and there's a sense of anxiety constantly hovering over us. That relationship, that work situation, that political situation, that traffic jam, those family members. It feels like they are all conspiring against us. It's that *When it rains, it pours* thinking.

We know that negative spirals go nowhere, and when we learn to manage our mind, we can start healing the brain and body! This kind of brain damage is reversible because the brain is neuroplastic: it can change, it always changes, and it's never too late to change. You can regenerate your brain.

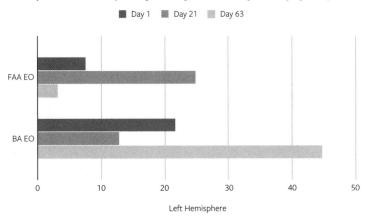

Subject 2: Frontal Alpha Asymmetry and Beta Asymmetry Eyes Open

■ Day 1 ■ Day 21 ▨ Day 63

Left Hemisphere

Changes in alpha and beta activity, based on qEEG data, over the course of study for this control subject. Alpha activity increases at day 21 on the left side of the brain. This indicates this subject is stuck in a thinking pattern of detail to the big picture. We see by day 63 this type of thinking has led to a large increase in beta activity on the left side of the brain, which is consistent with the red brain on the qEEG head map.

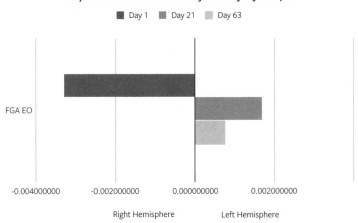

Subject 2: Frontal Gamma Asymmetry Eyes Open

■ Day 1 ■ Day 21 ▨ Day 63

Right Hemisphere   Left Hemisphere

Changes in gamma activity, based on qEEG data, over the course of study for this control subject. Gamma activity switches from the right hemisphere to the left hemisphere, suggesting again that this subject is stuck in detail to big picture thinking. We also see much less gamma activity at days 21 and 63 compared to day 1, suggesting that this person is not learning and changing.

Looking at the line graph for gamma activity in this subject in the figure below, we see that there is a very low "gamma peak," indicating that learning is not taking place and that the subject is suppressing their thoughts and not changing.

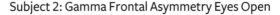

Subject 2: Gamma Frontal Asymmetry Eyes Open

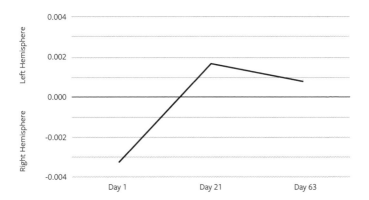

The line graph for gamma activity for the same control subject. As in the bar graph, we see gamma activity switch from the right hemisphere to the left hemisphere (negative values to positive values) but we do not see the "gamma peak" that is associated with learning and then solidifying the learning to form a habit.

In this control subject's brain, we observed a pattern of high beta activity in the dorsolateral prefrontal cortex (DLPFC), which increased over the course of the study. The DLPFC is an area that becomes active when we're making decisions, judgments, reacting emotionally, and reflecting. Too much activity here means you're not doing any of these things very well and impulsivity increases, which is exactly what the subject reported. They felt like they were making poor judgments, overreacting emotionally, and reflecting in a destructive way. They also felt like they were becoming increasingly negative and nothing made them happy.

This overactivity across these two areas also reflects a disconnect between the amygdala (emotional library) and the DLPFC (decisions and judgments). This means that the correct perceptions in the perceptual library of the amygdala cannot be accessed by the DLPFC, which loses out on this wise input because the toxic mindsets are dominating the person's thinking. This will have a negative effect on decision-making, switching attention, working memory, maintaining abstract rules, and inhibiting inappropriate responses. Picture a whole pile of books falling on top of you from the bookshelves in a library because you were trying to get too many down at once—that's what was happening in the subject's brain, contributing to their anxiety and affecting their ability to think clearly and with cognitive flexibility.

The subject's telomere length (DNA health), which shortened throughout the course of the study, also tells us more about the story playing out in the subject's brain and body—that they were getting increasingly unhealthy and putting themself at a higher risk for illness.

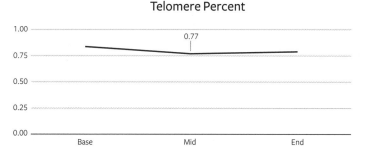

Telomere Percent

Telomere length in the control subject at three points of the study. This shows a change in telomere length from 84 percent at the beginning of the study to 79 percent by day 63. Typically, telomere length changes over years rather than weeks, suggesting that this control subject's lack of mind-management strategy may actually be shortening their life span at an alarming rate.

This subject was battling with underlying anguish, that nagging feeling that something is wrong. This was affecting their deep, non-REM sleep, which in turn was adding to their anxiety. From the data we observed, these sleep issues also affected their telomeres, which were shorter than they should have been, suggesting that their biological age was significantly older than their chronological age.

When we go into deep, regenerative sleep, we see a lot of delta waves in the brain, and at a certain frequency point when sleeping, the enzyme telomerase and growth hormone are released, which work with the telomeres to keep our cells healthy. This is an extremely important process, because we make around 810,000 cells every second and need strong, healthy telomere activity to do this.[3] The growth hormone, among many other things, helps with neuroplasticity. Delta waves should reduce during the day, but in this subject remained very high, indicating undealt-with and suppressed thoughts leading to feelings of hovering anxiety.

More on Millennials

Over the past several decades, in both my clinical practice and my research, I've observed an alarmingly noticeable increase in mental distress among Millennials, especially as they enter the workforce and try to make their way in life. In the clinical trial, we observed that the Millennials in the study appeared to fare worse when it came to dealing with stress compared to other generations.[4] Our analysis of the data showed that this age group is particularly susceptible to the effects of unmanaged chronic toxic stress and acute stress. There appears to be a correlation between the negative effects of toxic stress and the potential lack of mind-management within all demographics, but Millennials were especially suffering.

Why? Uncontrolled, toxic thinking has the potential to create a state of low-grade inflammation across the body and brain, affecting cortisol levels, hormones, brain functionality, and even telomeres on the chromosomes, as we discussed earlier. This creates a toxic feedback loop between the mind and the brain and body, activating the "hamster wheel" of toxic thinking, feeling, and choosing.

This is true across the board, but why are Millennials having such bad luck? Many of them are facing physical and mental burnout at a young age and at alarming rates. There are a variety of factors that could be contributing to this problem, but a few are highly competitive work and living environments (without the opportunities previous generations had, and with little hope for the future), extreme living costs and unequal wealth distribution, increased isolation, and a narrow focus on what they don't have alongside the desire for instant gratification—due, in large part, to social media, which may also be causing more issues with self-esteem and increased self-contempt. In fact, the instant universe that social media has created, which allows us to share information at lightning speeds without necessarily utilizing the tools and knowledge this information brings, has also led to many unrealistic expectations among people of all ages, and may be making Millennials unhappier and more anxious. These are just a few issues Millennials must deal with daily, and they're having a dramatic effect; despair and lower levels of well-being are playing a key role in fueling premature death in this age group.

Another possible reason Millennials are more adversely affected could be the increasing awareness and conversation around mental health struggles that's dominant in media, and other communication aimed at this age group, even though little or no effective and sustainable tools or techniques are presented to address the root causes. Though scaremongering may get good ratings, it can leave many people feeling hopeless and alone.

Indeed, few Millennials have been taught how to deal with making stress work for them, how to manage their mental health, or basic mind-management skills. Our society overemphasizes physical self-care, such as diet, exercise, and sleep (which are important but not the whole picture), to the exclusion of mind-management. When it comes to our happiness—we have pills for that, right?

Success and Happiness

There's a desperate need to teach people of all ages how to define their own success and happiness by *managing day-to-day life in a sustainable way*. We need to go beyond motivational catchphrases, mindfulness, medications, and pursuing happiness in an individualistic way to a deeper, more sustainable understanding of mind-management. We need to develop our sense of spirit— the resilient self-awareness that embodies our truth value, beliefs, values, passions, and meaning.

This isn't just a motivational speech. This is more than possible. I have observed, time and again, how people who have been taught to tune in to their nonconscious mind to manage their thought life and detox and build the brain, directing their neuroplasticity on a daily basis, are better able to navigate the ups and downs of life because they have a sense of control, which gives them hope—the pathway to empowerment, as I mentioned earlier. They embrace and process through situations—they see the light at the end through the tears and pain. They get forward momentum. They define their own path to success, notwithstanding societal constraints, physical impediments, or past traumas.

In our clinical trial, I saw this happening. The general trend across the experimental group, whose members were trained in mind-management, was one of progressive improvement, increased peace, and well-being. They learned how to manage their minds using the 5 Steps in a constructive, self-regulated way, which was reflected in the energy, connectivity, coherence, and balance observed in the brain, and the improvement in stress hormones and DNA, specifically telomeres. It was also evident in their narrative, where they described feeling more able to deal with barriers, challenges, and toxic stress on a daily basis.

This was, however, not the case for the control group, whose members didn't get the Neurocycle app. They experienced a worsening of self-regulated well-being, as reflected in the disturbed energy levels in the brain; poor connectivity, incoherence, and imbalance in the brain; and a worsening of stress hormones, homocysteine, and DNA, specifically telomeres. For the control group, the increased mindfulness that came from the measures applied in the study made them worse, because they didn't have a way of managing what they were becoming aware of.

> We need to become aware and empowered to manage what we become aware of.

The key takeaway here is that we need to become aware *and* empowered to manage what we become aware of. Empowerment comes through competency, which comes from having self-regulated, systematic steps and the know-how to apply the knowledge we have gained.

How Does This Help You?

The brain and body don't lie. They reflect what we're thinking, doing, and experiencing. The gut-brain interaction is one of the most obvious examples of this—most of us have experienced the impact shocking news has on our stomachs or in the ache of our hearts. This is why any kind of successful doing has to be supported by embracing the uncertainty you face in all its scariness and ambiguity, because inside this is the solution, the way forward—you can't move on until you're honest about where you are. You may think you can suppress your thoughts without consequences, but this is unfortunately not the case.

Your brain cannot change until you accept the anxiety or depression as a signal giving you information on its cause, or origin, and in this way you make the anxiety or depression work for you and not against you. This isn't necessarily clear-cut; your journey will be as unique as you are. The subjects in the experimental group recognized this and began developing increased self-regulation through using the 5 Steps, learning how to navigate and manage this new knowledge. The subjects in the control group, on the other hand, resorted to suppressing their issues because they felt disempowered and overwhelmed by their awareness of their issues—it was too much. We need to know *and manage* what we know.

Uncertainty

Uncertainty stimulates us to rise to the challenge. It compels us to look inward, accepting and embracing our discomfort even while not knowing what it brings—examining, wondering, asking, answering, discussing. We saw this happening in the experimental group, which is why I used the example of the "blue" depressed brain earlier (the "Subject 1 qEEG Z Scores" color image).

The 5 Steps of the Neurocycle give you a way to mind-manage with confidence both uncertainty and the unknown, which can help you face your issues and deal with them in a constructive and sustainable way. As you use them in your life to manage your thinking, you'll find that immensely trying times can have hidden dimensions you may miss if you don't accept all of the uncertainties! This is often when breakthroughs happen—when you don't understand something, your mind works extra hard to come up with a solution, which takes you to new levels of thinking.

This involves the hard work of digging into your nonconscious mind and getting comfortable with the uncomfortable so you can start seeing your breakdowns as good. You can use them to reconceptualize your toxic thoughts and trauma.

Here are some bonus tips on how to deal with the pain of uncertainty:

- Talk to someone you trust; having a friend makes things a little less scary.
- Balance out the uncertainty by focusing on what is certain.
- Repeat this mantra: "Things are uncertain, but I can handle it. I've never experienced this before, but I can handle it. These are uncertain times, but I can handle it. I have no idea what's going to happen, but I can handle it."

We can get ourselves into serious cycles of rumination and worry (the red brain discussed earlier) if we refuse to face our issues head-on and we don't progress forward. Going around and around and never making any progress leads to loads of anxiety. If we don't transform our pain through reconceptualization, we will transmit it, and it can then take over our thinking and our relationships. We need to reflect on the experiences we are going through in such a way that we accept that even though we may not be able to make sense of them, we can still deal with them—and move forward.

So many times we get stuck looking for *why* someone did something because it feels like that's where our peace will come from. We think, *If I only knew their reason for doing what they did.* Unfortunately, often we cannot understand others' actions or why so many things go wrong at once—we aren't experts on other people's motives or experiences; we're only experts on ourselves. In trying to make sense of them, we often see the actions and words of others through the lens of our own experiences, but we can never really know what another person is thinking, and we may never be able to make sense of the pain they caused us in the way we want to. And these thoughts will only keep us stuck in the pain.

> It is in the breakdown that we break down toxic thoughts, habits, and trauma.

Accepting uncertainty may be how you finally find peace about a situation, which can reduce your anxiety and allow you to move on. In our clinical trial, as the subjects in the experimental group started coming to grips with their issues, we saw changes in the nonconscious mind reflected in the brain. Throughout the study we saw an increase in the alpha wave activity, which is often referred to as the *alpha bridge*, because it reflects the bridging between the nonconscious mind and the conscious mind. Alpha increases when we choose to tune in to our thoughts and face our issues, which means the brain is calming down as well.

If we're empowered mentally, we put our peace and happiness in our own hands. I see this all the time in my research, clinical practice, and the response I get from my audiences. As I said at the beginning of this book, true transformation requires mind-management strategies to rewire neural pathways. Directing the way your brain changes—using mind-management to direct neuroplasticity—changes energy patterns in the brain, changes our blood measures, and eventually establishes a new and healthy level of balance in the brain and body.

The preliminary results of this study suggest that the subjects who used the Neurocycle app daily as part of their mind-management strategy were learning to read the signals, embrace them, identify the cause of their depression and/or anxiety and burnout, and manage their mind on a daily basis (as a lifestyle strategy). They were making their depression and anxiety work for them and not against them. They learned how to use their *conscious* mind to tune in and connect with the warning signals in their *subconscious* mind, which enabled them to find the thought pattern they wanted to deal with in the *nonconscious* mind. They were processing their thoughts and learning how to reconceptualize them. Through this simple, proactive approach of the Neurocycle they were able to direct the neuroplasticity of their brain in a therapeutic way. They were on the path to empowerment!

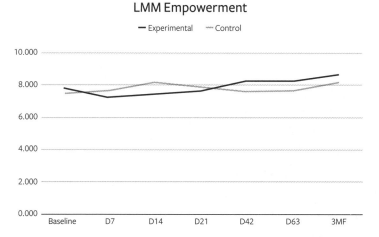

Change in empowerment over time during the study between the control group and the experimental group. We see a trend toward increasing empowerment in the experimental group, which was sustained at six months after the study was completed. This suggests that the new habits formed in the experimental group were sustainable over time, confirming the persistence of neuroplastic changes. The control group, however, showed less empowerment compared to the experimental group by the end of the study.

Depression and anxiety are highly correlated with burnout, so we'd expect to see a reduction in anxiety leading to burnout if depression and anxiety are managed. The subjects in the experimental group reported this in their narrative, and we also observed this trend in the psychological scales. We also saw these positive trends correlating with changes in their neuroendocrine hormones, the HPA axis, and their genes, specifically the telomeres, which are all strong indicators of how well toxic stress is being managed.

How Does This Help You?

Once again, true transformation requires mind-management strategies to rewire neural pathways. Directing the way your brain changes (neuroplasticity) transforms energy patterns in the brain, changes blood measures, and eventually establishes a new and healthy level of balance in the brain and body. You, like the study subjects, can use the Neurocycle to methodically use your mind to take advantage of neuroplasticity to rework your neural circuitry, managing and improving a variety of mental and physical states, even if you have very dysfunctional brain networks and physiology from toxic thoughts and trauma.

> True transformation requires mind-management strategies to rewire neural pathways.

The path to empowerment is not only attainable but within you! *You* can guide and direct changes in your brain. The 5 Steps will not only empower you to push through the pain that may come from the healing work, but will also give you a structured, scientifically researched, and effective process that works and a defined time period for the process, which will further reduce your pain and uncertainty and make the process more effective and sustainable.

If these 5 Steps are utilized to make mental health care more easily accessible and applicable to everyone, regardless of circumstances, then I know I have accomplished my life mission.

These 5 Steps have helped me turn my life around from being in a mental hospital because of attempted suicide to actually facing the trauma that got me there and coming to like myself as a person. I have learned that I can be in control and don't have to be a victim to my own thoughts.

HALEY

Chapter 6

What Is the Mind?

Man can alter his life by altering his thinking.
WILLIAM JAMES

Overview

- Your mind is not your brain, just as you are not your brain.
- When you think, you will feel, and when you think and feel, you will choose. These three aspects always work together. This is the mind-in-action.
- A thought itself is the concept, the big idea. Thoughts have memories, like trees have branches. There are three types of memories in a thought: information, emotions, and physical sensations.
- Thoughts are located in three different places: in your brain, in the cells of your body, and in your mind.
- During the day you think, feel, and choose to *build* new thoughts into your mind and brain; at night you think, feel, and choose to *sort out* the thoughts you have built during the day, which provides the content for dreams.
- Self-regulation is the overarching catalyst of successful mind-management—and is your brain's favorite exercise! When we don't self-regulate, we will suffer mentally and physically.

What is the mind? It can be a tricky concept, so it's best to start with what the mind is not. Your mind is *not* your brain, just as you are not your brain. The mind is separate, yet inseparable from, the brain. The mind uses the brain, and the brain responds to the mind. The brain doesn't produce the mind. The mind changes the brain. People do things; our brains do not force us to do things. Yes, there would be no conscious experience without the brain, but experience cannot be reduced to the brain's actions.

The mind is energy, and it generates energy through thinking, feeling, and choosing. That means we generate energy through our mind-in-action 24/7, which is part of the activity we pick up with brain technology. When we generate this mind energy through thinking, feeling, and choosing, we build thoughts, which are physical structures in our brain. This building of thoughts is called *neuroplasticity*.

In our clinical trials, we saw how the energy in the brain changed as the subject was thinking and how this stimulated neuroplasticity; the brain was responding to the person's thinking, feeling, and choosing as a stream of consciousness and nonconscious activity. The mind is a stream of *nonconscious* and *conscious* activity when we're awake, and a stream of *nonconscious* activity when we're asleep. It's characterized by a triad of thinking, feeling, and choosing. When you think, you will feel, and when you think and feel, you will choose. These three aspects always work together.

The conscious mind is awake when you're awake and is limited in what it can pay attention to. The nonconscious mind is awake and working 24/7 and is huge and infinite. The subconscious mind is between the two, kind of like that tip-of-the-tongue feeling. The unconscious mind is when you're knocked out or under anesthetic.

You have a unique way you think, feel, and choose, which is your *identity*. When your thinking, feeling, and choosing are off for some reason, this will affect your identity.

When you think, feel, and choose, you create, and this creation is a *thought*. And you're always thinking, feeling, and choosing. When you're awake, you think and feel and choose to build thoughts. When you're asleep, you sort out the thoughts you've built during the day.

What does the brain have to do with all of this? The brain is an extremely complex neuroplastic responder. This essentially means that each time it's stimulated by your mind, it responds in many different ways, including neurochemical, genetic, and electromagnetic changes. This, in turn, grows and changes structures in the brain, building or wiring in new physical thoughts. The brain is never the same because it changes with every experience you have, every moment of every day—and you control this with your unique thinking, feeling, and choosing. You use your mind to use your brain. You are the architect of your brain.

What's in a Thought?

The mind is made up of trillions and trillions of thoughts. A thought is a *real physical thing* that occupies mental real estate in the brain and mind. A thought is built into the brain as you use your mind—that is, as you think and feel and choose. Thoughts look like trees. We say in neuroscience that a thought has an arbor-like structure. Look at the three images below to see the tree-like structure of thoughts.

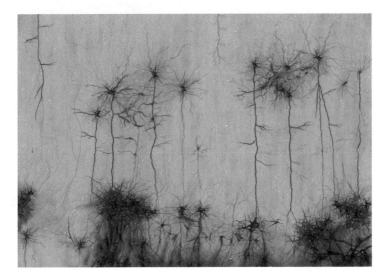

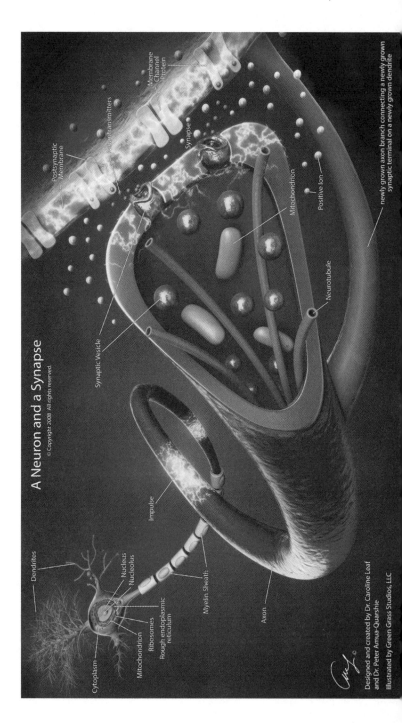

A Neuron and a Synapse

Dendrites

Nucleus
Nucleolus

Cytoplasm

Mitochondrion
Ribosomes
Rough endoplasmic
reticulum

Myelin Sheath

Impulse

Axon

Synaptic Vesicle

Postsynaptic
Membrane

Neurotransmitters

Membrane
Channel
Protein

Synapse

Mitochondrion

Positive Ion

Neurotubule

newly grown axon branch connecting a newly grown
synaptic terminal on a newly grown dendrite

Designed and created by Dr. Caroline Leaf
and Dr. Peter Amua-Quarshie
Illustrated by Green Grass Studios, LLC

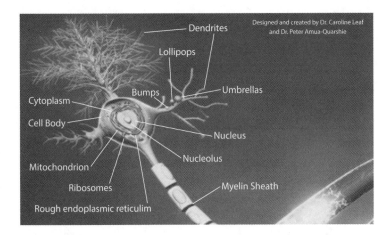

A thought itself is the concept, the big idea. Inside the thought are the embedded memories—so a thought is made of memories, and there can be any number of memories, thousands even, in a thought, just as there are hundreds or even thousands of branches on a tree. For example, the thought could be *I am concerned about my family member.* Within this thought, there will be hundreds or more memories related to this concern. The thought is therefore the big picture, and the details of the thought are the memories.

There are three types of memories in a thought:

1. **Informational memories** are all the details: particulars, facts, data, associations, links, and so on associated with that thought. These are like the branches on a thought tree.

2. **Emotional memories** are the feelings associated with the information memories. These are like the leaves on the branches of a thought three.

3. **Physical memories** are the physical embodiments of the sensations experienced at the time the thought was built, which are coupled with the emotional memories and informational memories. These are built into every cell of our body and are reexperienced when we recall the

information and feeling memories, because these three parts of the thought are inseparable.

The image below, the thought tree, is an analogy for the anatomy of a thought. As I mentioned above, a thought is the big concept: the whole tree with branches, leaves, and roots. The branches and leaves are *how* you express your memories as your *conscious* thinking, feeling, and choosing, which produce your behaviors and your communication (what you are saying and doing) and all of which manifest your lifestyle choices. The tree trunk represents the *subconscious* level and your perspective, which includes the physical and emotional signals you experience, such as that lurch of anticipation when you hear exciting news, that sense of happiness or joy that makes you bounce out of bed, or that nagging sense of depression or anxiety that something is wrong. The subconscious connects the nonconscious to the conscious, in the same way the trunk connects the roots to the leaves and branches. The roots represent the *nonconscious* roots of your memories. They are the origin of the informational, emotional, and physical memories and are the level that tells us what's going on in our lives and why we do what we do—this is the level we have to tap into to make

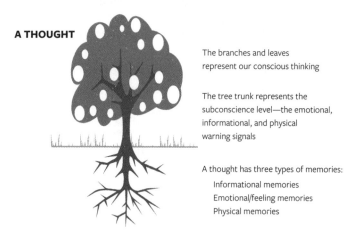

A THOUGHT

The branches and leaves represent our conscious thinking

The tree trunk represents the subconscience level—the emotional, informational, and physical warning signals

A thought has three types of memories:
Informational memories
Emotional/feeling memories
Physical memories

the changes needed in our lifestyles, and the level into which the 5 Steps are designed to tap.

In the same way that a planted seed forms roots, appears above ground, grows, and changes, so your thoughts grow and change over time. Once a thought is planted—the conversation you have, what you hear, what you read, and so on—its roots begin to grow. When "watered" with thinking, it grows into a little thought plant. If ignored, the thought tree dies. If, however, it gets lots of thinking energy, it will eventually get bigger and stronger. Whatever we think about the most will grow. So, at first it is a little plant, like a nagging worry or something at the back of your mind. Over time, if it's watered with thinking, it becomes a "big tree" and can dominate and influence our behavior.

To detox a toxic thought, we first observe our behaviors and emotions, which show us the branches and leaves on the thought tree. Then we look at our perspective, or our mind-in-action. We see this perspective by tuning in to the emotional and physical warning signals we experience, such as anxiety, depression, a sore gut, or aching muscles. The subconscious warning signals (the tree trunk) take us deeper into the nonconscious to see informational and emotional memories (the cause or origin) and to build the root.

The exciting thing is that *you* are the director and designer of this process! You shape what you have built, and you can change what is not working or what is having a negative effect in your life. Toxic thought trees like trauma and bad habits can be built and broken down and rebuilt—toxic trees aren't your destiny.

This is self-regulated mind-management. Your thinking, feeling, and choosing are shaping, pruning, and building. And the more self-regulated you are, the more effective this process is and the more peace and meaning you'll find in life.

How Many Thoughts Do We Think in a Day?

Thoughts are potentially limitless. Each thought is a literal universe, because each thought is made up of limitless memories. Thoughts also keep getting updated, as well as entangled with other related thoughts, like the endless root system of a sweeping forest. And your mind is always in action, which means you're always building thoughts. And you're always pulling up the thoughts you have built to guide and influence your next decision.

Just think of how much information you're being exposed to in any one moment, hour, day, week, month, and year of your life! From the moment you wake up, you're getting new information about your environment, your relationships, your work, your community, and the wider world. You view this information through your unique way of thinking, feeling, and choosing—your unique lens through which you see and interact with the world. This means you're always in the process of adding new memories to your existing thoughts.

So, how many thoughts do we actually *think* in a day? The answer is complicated because we're always building new memories into our existing thoughts; building entirely new thoughts with their embedded informational, emotional, and physical memories in response to information from our environment (from people, what we read, what we see, and so on); and pulling up existing thoughts. We're also building new thoughts as we daydream and as our minds wander.

According to anesthesiologist and researcher Professor Stuart Hamerhoff, we have conscious bursts of activity around forty times a second, which is our thinking, feeling, and choosing, or our mind-in-action.[1] We experience these bursts like a cartoon strip, where all the individual frames are experienced as a conscious event about every ten seconds, somewhat similar to watching an animated movie.

Each individual frame is a thought, with thousands of embedded memories. However, we aren't conscious of all the detailed memories in these frames at these time points, just the big-picture concept of the thought. For example, in the time it took me to type this sentence I have had forty conscious bursts of activity. As I continue to type and explain this concept, I have hit the ten-second mark, and have just had a conscious event where I realized I had five other random thoughts pop into my conscious mind. I didn't focus on any of these because I am writing this book, so they sank back into my nonconscious mind, while the next few popped up. And so the cycle continues. We have an estimated six of these conscious bursts per minute, around 360 per hour (6 x 60), and 8,460 every twenty-four hours (360 x 24).

On the nonconscious level, it's a whole different story: intelligent thinking occurs at about a *million* operations per second, and general brain activity occurs at about 10^{27} operations per second.[2] Thoughts with their embedded memories that have sufficient energy will move into the conscious mind at a rate of about five to seven approximately every five to ten seconds, sometimes quicker, which equals around eight thousand thoughts every twenty-four hours.[3] Totaling the thoughts from external signals and the internal thoughts together, we have anything from an estimated sixteen to eighteen thousand thoughts each day.

Even though it's interesting to conjecture about numbers, as it can help us understand how important it is to control what we let into our heads as well as control what's already there, we should not get too hung up about them. Instead, we should focus on the *enormity of the power of our nonconscious mind* and learn how to use that power more effectively through mind-management.

It's also important to remember that although our thought-life is a stream of consciousness, with thousands of individual thoughts blending together, we can bring a level of order to our thinking by controlling what we allow into our mind and brain and what's already in our mind and brain. We're able to evaluate the individual frames of thought by self-regulating our stream of consciousness. We can harness the power of our thinking in tangible, sustainable ways.

Where Are Thoughts Located?

Thoughts are located in three different places: in your brain, in your mind, and in the cells of your body.

The Brain

Thoughts with their embedded memories are stored physically in the brain as energy vibrations in protein supercomputers, called *tubulin*, in the dendrites on your neurons.[4] As we think, feel, and choose, we grow more dendrites into the brain for the new memories, which are added to existing thoughts in a reconceptualized, redesigned way. Each update reconfigures the entire thought with a new perspective because it's an organic, dynamic system, and the whole perspective of the thought changes.

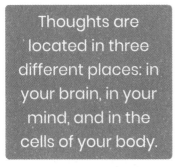

Thoughts are located in three different places: in your brain, in your mind, and in the cells of your body.

The Mind

Thoughts with their embedded memories are also stored in the nonconscious mind as an energy field. This is the deep, spiritual level of a thought, which goes beyond the physical but is intimately connected to it.

This spiritual level of thought storage is about you and your truth value; that is, your unique perception and way of experiencing the world.

The Cells

The third place thoughts with their embedded memories are stored is in the cells of the body. Estimates of how many cells we have in our bodies range from fifty to one hundred trillion, while more recent studies indicate there are around thirty-seven trillion cells in our body.[5] Thoughts that are stored in our cells are called *cellular memory*.

An easy example to help understand these three places of thought storage is catching a virus. If you catch a virus, your immune system builds up antibodies so that if you get exposed to that virus again, the cells of your immune system remember and send out immune factors to fight this virus. These cells even embed how you were feeling physically at the time. For example, if you had a touch of the flu or a really sore stomach at the time you were experiencing something, you build this experience into the thought. When the thought is recalled, the informational memory (what happened, or the facts), emotions (feelings), and physical sensations (flu-like symptoms, sore stomach, and so on) come flooding back. Now you see why recalling thoughts, especially those of a traumatic nature, can literally make you sick.

Epigenetics

The vibrational frequency energy from the thoughts in the brain can be picked up by various brain technologies, like EEG and qEEG, which is what we used in our recent clinical trial. This energy is transmitted from the thought at quantum speeds (faster than 10^{27}) to all the cells of the body, literally bathing them in an energy that is either toxic, healthy, or neutral and creating a reaction in the brain and body, causing all kinds of chemicals, hormones, and electromagnetic responses to occur. For example, in our clinical trial, levels of cortisol and homocysteine increased more than they should in response to the toxic thoughts and stress of some of the subjects, and normalized when their toxic thoughts and stress were managed using the Neurocycle method.[6] Our thinking, feeling, and choosing change the thoughts *and the impact these thoughts have on the body*. This is called *epigenetics*.

Epigenetics is what switches the genes on and off. *Epi* means "above" or "over," so epigenetics is over and above the genes. As long as we're alive, genes are constantly being switched on and off by the mind and by what we put into and onto our body, which can be passed through the generations as predispositions. This works through chemical tags (the addition of a methyl or acetyl group, or a "chemical cap," to part of the DNA molecule) added to chromosomes that, in effect, switch genes on or off like turning a light on or off by pressing the switch.

Thoughts even impact to the level of the DNA and chromosomes in our cells. Our experiences change the gene structure and gene activity, not the gene sequence. In our research study, the subjects' thinking impacted changes in their telomere length (TL) and biological age.[7] The TL shortened when toxic thoughts affected cell health but increased with mind-management of toxic thoughts and toxic stress. Constantly recalling negative thoughts with their embedded memories can damage our DNA (shortened TL), which can create a vulnerability in our body to disease.[8] However, embracing, processing, and reconceptualizing thoughts with their embedded memories can heal damaged DNA (lengthened TL) and, by inference, decrease vulnerability to disease.

> *I am twenty-three and an Armenian born in Aleppo, Syria.*
> *As you might know, the war started in Syria, and in August*
> *2012 my family and I moved to Lebanon. Around that time*
> *many people were trying to go to Germany/Europe through*
> *Turkey with boats. On November 29 it was our turn to take*
> *the journey on a very small boat in the middle of the night. It*
> *was my dad, mom, grandma, little brother who had just turned*
> *ten, and me. In the middle of the journey, in the middle of the*
> *sea, the engine of the boat stopped, and a few minutes later*
> *the boat sank with my family trapped inside the small room.*
> *My dad and I were outside on the deck and we tried to swim*
> *to survive. It was freezing cold and so dark that I could barely*
> *see. A few minutes later I saw my dad's floating body near me.*

He couldn't survive the cold and the waves. I was there in the middle of the sea alone for a few hours. Life hasn't been easy for years. I loved my family so much, I felt so lost and weak for days. These 5 Steps and your research helped me through my everyday life and challenges. I still struggle but at least now I have a plan to manage my mind and help with healing.

ARINA

Chapter 7

The Interconnected Mind

Overview

- Whatever we think about the most grows, because we are giving it energy.
- The mind is divided into the conscious mind (fully aware when you are awake), the nonconscious mind (works 24/7), and the subconscious mind (just-aware level).
- We don't need to be held captive to our thoughts; instead, we can "capture" our thoughts.
- Whatever you experience in your mind will also be experienced in your brain and body. The toxic energy from toxic thoughts accumulates if it isn't dealt with, and will eventually explode, affecting the way we think, feel, and choose in a volcanic and uncontrolled way.
- Dealing with our toxic thoughts and traumas means that all this swirling, chaotic, toxic energy needs to be transferred from the negative thought to the reconceptualized, healthy thought to restore balance and coherence to the mind.

In learning about how to use our mind to manage our mind, it helps to understand the divisions of the mind and how these relate to the dynamic nature of thoughts. There are basically two ways of managing the mind: *reactively*, which generally ends up being messy, or *proactively*, which is how we clean up our mental mess. Developing a lifelong plan that helps you constantly manage thoughts and their impact is part of a proactive and strategic approach. You can even think of this as "preventative" medicine for your brain. The 5 Steps are how you do this, and they can teach you how to manage your mind proactively and strategically, facilitating optimal brain functioning that will allow you to get the best out of your brain by cleaning up your mental mess.

And, as you learn to manage your mind, you're doing some amazing things. For example, you're guiding how the energy moves through your brain and how this energy influences your body, including which genes switch on and off, the length of your telomeres, how the chemicals flow through your bloodstream, and controlling things like cortisol.

In this section, we're going to look a little deeper into the divisions of the mind to help you better understand your mind, which will equip you to mind-manage in the best way possible. When you understand the *why*, the *how* becomes so much easier.

The mind is divided into the conscious mind, the nonconscious mind, and the subconscious mind. Below is a table summarizing these divisions, followed by a discussion explaining these divisions and how they are relevant to learning how to manage your mind.

TABLE 3. The Divisions of the Mind

Conscious Mind	Fully aware, awake when we're awake, and functions best when we're deliberate, intentional, actively self-regulated, and proactive.
Subconscious Mind	"Just aware" level where thoughts move from the nonconscious to the conscious mind.
Nonconscious Mind	The swirling, high-energy powerhouse that works 24/7, where all memories are stored. It's our wisdom and intelligence. It involves a dynamic, self-regulated process that is the potent and effectual driving force behind our communication and behavior. It's always online working with the conscious when the conscious mind is awake. It's in constant conversation with the subconscious mind, working to bring balance and clean up our mental mess.

Unconscious Mind	This is not a division of the mind, per se, but rather something that can be *done* to your mind. When you get knocked out, for example, from a concussion, drinking too much, or being anesthetized for surgery, you become unconscious.

Let's look at another image of a thought tree, below, as an analogy for the divisions of the mind, which makes it easier to picture these divisions. The top of the tree is the conscious mind, which is our communication and behavior, or what we say and do. The tree trunk area and the grass are the subconscious mind, which are the prompts from the nonconscious mind that are just on the edge of our conscious awareness. These are those tip-of-the-tongue, can't-quite-put-your-finger-on-it cues that evoke and trigger that feeling that something needs to be addressed—something is trying to get our attention. The nonconscious mind is the deep spiritual and phenomenally fast quantum world where our truth value, intelligence, wisdom, meaning, and thoughts with their embedded memories are stored in a swirling mass of energy.

These three parts of mind, of which the nonconscious is the biggest, form about 90 to 99 percent of who you are. Your brain and body are about 1 percent of who you are. This is based on my

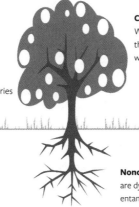

A THOUGHT

A thought is a concept and has three parts:

Informational memories
Emotional/feeling memories
Physical memories

Conscious mind = Fully aware state. Whatever we say and do comes from thoughts, which are the root of our words and actions.

Subconscious mind = Prompts from the nonconscious mind in the form of emotional, informational, and physical warning signals.

Nonconscious mind = Where thoughts are dynamically interacting and are entangled.

research and theory, The Geodesic Information Processing Theory, a summary of which is in appendix A.

When you consciously engage the nonconscious mind through deliberate, intentional, strategic, and proactive deep thinking, you draw your thoughts, with their embedded memories, through the subconscious mind and into the conscious mind. When these thoughts arrive in the conscious mind, they're in a malleable state, which means you can change them and reconceptualize them. You also tune in to the physical warning signals associated with how you feel, such as an increased heartrate, an adrenaline rush, a headache, or a stomachache. Next, you embrace any feelings, such as anxiety or depression, as an emotional warning signal that something is going on in your life.

Instead of seeing these as negative, you see them as telling you something: you make them work for you and not against you. You do this in a celebratory way, not because you're celebrating the painful memories but because *now you're conscious of them*, which means you can change them. Remember, you can change only what you are conscious of.

We have self-regulatory power when we're conscious, which is kind of like what Benjamin Libet famously called "veto power" over our thoughts.[1] This power allows you to control your thoughts. You can literally capture them and, using your self-regulatory veto power, change them. As you do this, you override the force generated from the energy of the toxic thought, and choose to speak or act, or not, according to this thought. You can even evaluate the thought and decide if you want to change it, when to change it, and how to change it. You don't have to be driven by toxic ruminations and reactions from established negative thought patterns or traumas, because you have the power to veto them. This is a proactive way of approaching the mind and can save you a lot of heartache and anxiety.

I'm sure you have already experienced this numerous times: you are just about to say or do something but stop yourself for some reason. Maybe you feel it's the wrong timing, or that the person is already upset and it would only make matters worse. This is mind-management in action, and one of the many ways we can clean up the mental mess.

In order to make changes in our thoughts and subsequent communication, we need to be strategic, proactive, and deliberate about our thinking. We need to make an effort to be aware of what we are thinking about every day. This is self-regulation, and it works hand in hand with our veto power. This is exciting! We don't need to be held captive to our thoughts; instead, we can capture our thoughts.

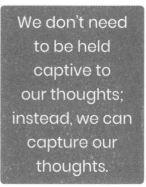

We don't need to be held captive to our thoughts; instead, we can capture our thoughts.

Deliberate, intentional, self-regulated thinking is key to good mind-management because it starts the downstream flow into the subconscious and nonconscious mind. Unfortunately, such thinking isn't a high priority in our hurry-sickness, consumer-driven technological world, where we just don't take the time. We don't like deep thinking in this era, and we're paying the price for it.

Why Is the Nonconscious Mind So Important?

The nonconscious mind is incredible but often misunderstood. Even the word *nonconscious* is used incorrectly most of the time. Yet it's worth putting in the effort to try to understand it, because it's a key player when it comes to mind-management. It's *definitely not* some preprogrammed tape on replay, making us operate like some kind of avatar, as it's often depicted.

My PhD theory, The Geodesic Information Processing Theory, was birthed out of research on the nonconscious mind, and all my research since has been to better understand, expand, and develop this theory in order to improve the mind-management techniques I've developed. My recent clinical trials demonstrate how nonconscious activity can be picked up by a qEEG and my psychological scale, the Leaf Mind-Management Scale (LMM). Although we can "fake it" on a conscious level, our nonconscious level always tells the truth about what's *actually* going on in our mind. You may think you can, but you can't lie to yourself, and you most definitely won't get away with it, because your brain and body carry the effects of the lie.

> We get valuable little packets of information in the form of emotional and physical warning signals around every ten seconds.

If you're going to learn how to manage your mind, you have to train yourself to think in a way that taps into your nonconscious intelligence. The conscious mind lags behind the nonconscious mind by at least ten seconds, so it takes about ten seconds before you're consciously aware of what's going on—and it's roughly in this ten seconds that the truth of the situation will try to get your attention through emotional and physical warning signals.[2]

So, we get valuable little packets of information in the form of emotional and physical warning signals around every ten seconds, and the more we train ourselves to tune in, the more we can discern and use these signals to control our reactions. You may not get all the details straightaway, but as you push through, over the 63-day cycle we'll learn in part 2, little by little these signals will be revealed to you as information is constantly updated. The 5 Steps will help train you to tune in to your nonconscious mind.

As we talked about earlier, in our clinical trials we analyzed different types of psychological data using a number of scales traditionally used to diagnose and label someone as clinically depressed or anxious. These scales show how someone was reacting in that moment but not how they were functioning mentally over time. If, for example, you had to go to the hospital for a surgery, you would definitely be feeling a combination of anxiety and depression, but this doesn't necessarily mean you have clinical anxiety or depression. Rather, you're having a very normal reaction to an adverse circumstance. You don't need your misery medicalized or your pain pathologized. You need to be listened to. Yet these scales are used to determine someone's mental state, which can be scary considering the implications of many current treatments, which are predominantly drug-based with a number of long-term side effects, and the stigmatization that's often associated with mental health labels.

However, using the scientifically validated mind-management scale I developed, the LMM, and the person's narrative and qEEG measures, we were able to get a much clearer and more realistic picture of what was going on in the subjects' minds. Instead of being labeled as clinically depressed or anxious, the subjects in the study learned that the mental chaos on the nonconscious level

> With mind-management, we can start seeing that depression and anxiety are coming from normal reactions to the experiences of life.

in the mind was operating like a nonconscious driver, pushing through the subconscious level to the conscious level. They learned to experience these prompts from the nonconscious mind as emotional and physical warning signals, telling them something was up and needed attention.

These prompts were things like depression, anxiety, angst, frustration, edginess, irritability, and so on, and were normal reactions to what they were going through. Once they started working on them, subjects started *seeing* they were coming from normal reactions to the experiences of life, including traumatic, suppressed life events such as childhood abuse. By day 21, the depression, anxiety, and so on had lifted dramatically in the experimental group, who were using the 5 Steps of mind-management. They felt like they were back online, functioning better at work and in their relationships, and sleeping better, to mention just a few things. This improvement was sustained and getting better by day 63, indicating that the 5 Steps were helping the subjects clean up their mental mess.

> The more you understand the nonconscious mind, the more you will see that you also have the ability to **change** your mind.

The more you understand the nonconscious mind, the more you will see that you also have the ability to *change* your mind. The nonconscious mind has often been confused with the subconscious and unconscious mind and relegated to a kind of fancy storage cabinet for mechanistic-style programs that run our conscious actions. However, the nonconscious mind is far more than that. It's a swirling, organized aggregation of energy, hungry for change, growth, learning, and order and filled with wisdom. When you think about it, you know what you can handle, and this is your nonconscious mind's wisdom. At your core, you are *wisdom*. The nonconscious mind hates operating in chaos and disequilibrium. This high-energy powerhouse works 24/7, and it's where all our thoughts are stored as living, buzzing masses of energy just waiting to be transferred to the conscious mind to propel us into action.

Intelligent thinking happens at about a million actions per second in the nonconscious mind. The general activity that is going on 24/7, which is part of us just being alive, operates at 10^{27}. This is a blow-your-mind kind of speed, way faster than the speed of light. It makes sense though, because the speed that electrical activity fires throughout the neurons in the brain is too slow to account for the speed at which thoughts impact the brain and the body, so we have to turn to quantum physics (which explains the speed of energy in the nonconscious mind) to understand how we get from A to B. Logically, whatever you experience in your mind will also be experienced in your brain and body. There's a plethora of research dating back many years on the mind-body connection; it's even spoken about in ancient texts. Our nonconscious mind expresses itself through the brain and body, which can be picked up with qEEG readings.

The nonconscious mind is characterized by a dynamic, self-regulated process that's a high-powered, potent, and effectual driving force behind our communication and behavior; that is, everything we say and do, mixing and matching our beliefs, views, and experiences (memories inside thoughts) with our incoming experiences to help make sense of the world. It's always online, working with the conscious mind when we are awake. It's that perception, that assumption, those implicit biases, that way we view the world; it's involved in supplying information we need as we make decisions; it's everywhere in everything all the time. It's in constant conversation with the subconscious and conscious mind, working to bring balance and clean up our mental mess.

These conversations come out in our dreams, in those hovering feelings of anxiety or angst, or in the signals of depression, happiness, and anger we experience. And it's not just the negative that the nonconscious wants to push into our conscious mind to get sorted out to restore equilibrium. The nonconscious mind is more focused on the good stuff, like our happiness, excitement, joy, and passion. When we sense these feelings subconsciously, we should capture them and focus on them, because they put the brain into a resilient state that allows higher levels of learning to take place, and we can operate judiciously. Humor, empathy, and gratitude also help us do this—all these good values are like the ingredients of wisdom and resilience in our nonconscious mind and are just waiting to be used to help us operate at a higher level.

This is why the nonconscious mind is often seen as our "spiritual" level and is the most extensive and influential part of the mind. It's very attuned to keeping us mentally and physically healthy, so as soon as we have toxic thoughts, which come with a lot of toxic energy attached to them that upsets the equilibrium in the nonconscious mind, it will send us warning signals such as depression and anxiety, or that nagging sense that something is wrong.

Much like a small child that has been kept indoors for too long and when let outside is like a ball of energy being released, these pent-up signals can often manifest themselves in physical symptoms such as tight muscles, whooshes of adrenaline, headaches, and GI symptoms. As soon as these physical and emotional warning signals come into our subconscious mind, they're prompting us to listen up, saying, *There's a thought issue going on here that needs some conscious attention!* We need to learn to listen to these signals and understand them by getting in touch with our nonconscious mind, because it holds the power to clean up our mental space.

> When we become deliberate, intentional, self-regulated thinkers, we tune in to the subconscious mind, which takes us deeper into the nonconscious mind.

The nonconscious mind also monitors the emotional balance in our mental and physical space, always striving for coherence between the different parts of the mind. As mentioned above, it does that by prompting the conscious mind, sending the high-energy healthy or toxic thoughts to the subconscious mind. When we become deliberate, intentional, self-regulated thinkers, we tune in to the subconscious mind, which takes us deeper into the nonconscious mind. That's how we draw out our problematic toxic habits or the traumas that are draining our mental and physical energy, which is the first step to dealing with them. We balance the toxic energy with the positive energy as we embrace, process, and reconceptualize our thoughts.

It's important to remember that throughout this process energy is never lost but rather always transferred—this is a basic law of physics. Toxic energy creates a messy disturbance in the brain, which results in an imbalance in the nonconscious mind. That, in turn, creates an imbalance in the brain that will be picked up by a qEEG (remember the red and blue head maps?). This toxic energy accumulates if it isn't dealt with, and will eventually explode, affecting our mind-in-action in a volcanic and uncontrolled way.

This toxic energy needs to get transferred from the nonconscious to the subconscious and then to the conscious mind. I'm sure you have experienced this in some way in your life. For example, you just get so angry and are so tired of someone behaving the way they do that you say or do some very ugly things; you break down and just can't deal with it anymore. Volcanic explosions can be experienced as breakdowns, extreme anxiety, depression, OCD, PTSD, psychotic breaks, mounting frustration, a sense of sadness that doesn't ever seem to go away, a physical illness, or a mixture of these, called *comorbidity*. Everyone will experience these explosions in different ways and for different periods of time, because our experiences, and the way we experience these experiences, are unique. The good news is that when we embrace these signals from the nonconscious, we can do something about them before they cause more physical and mental problems.

Dealing with our toxic thoughts and traumas means that all this swirling, chaotic, toxic energy needs to be transferred from the negative thought to the reconceptualized, healthy thought in order to restore balance and coherence to the mind. Essentially, our nonconscious mind is like a first-class housekeeper: it's always looking for toxic disturbances, rooting them out, and dropping hints into the subconscious mind through emotional and physical warning signals.

The toxic thought is then transferred into the conscious mind, where we gather awareness of it. What this means is that the gatherer (you) needs to draw the toxic thought into the conscious mind. Once it's in the conscious mind, directed neuroplasticity kicks in, and the protein branches holding the memory information in vibrational frequencies weaken. That's when the thought is at its weakest and can be reconceptualized, which is why I keep talking about *embracing our issues*: we need to face them and become aware of them—that is, be conscious of them—by gathering an awareness of the signals in our subconscious mind. Once we do this, we can draw out the toxic stuff in our nonconscious mind and bring it into the conscious mind, where it's weakened and malleable. Only then can we process and reconceptualize this mindset and move forward. It's hard and sometimes very painful, but in our weakness, we can find strength.

It's also important to remember that drawing out toxic thoughts isn't the only thing the nonconscious mind is good for. It's also where we find intelligent insight (those *aha* moments), get discernment, and are able to be judicious and logical about any given situation. It's the source of our rationale, foresight, and hindsight. So, as we tune in to the nonconscious mind, we can make use of all this good stuff.

> Through the nonconscious mind, we can access good thoughts as well as toxic thoughts.

There's also another part to our relationship with the nonconscious mind. Through it, we can access our good thoughts and use these in a multitude of ways, such as remembering a good time with a loved one to help calm down or deal with grief, recalling a time when we got through a challenge to encourage ourselves to press forward, and remembering vital information for a test we studied hard for. All thoughts with their informational and emotional memories can be reconsolidated when we're conscious of them; that is, when we recall them from the nonconscious mind. And when the memories go back into the nonconscious mind, they're always more complex than before, like adding another layer to a painting. You don't simply add more information to the thought, nor do you try to cancel it out with another thought. Rather, you redesign the memories in the thought to be less painful and more manageable. Your story is included in the new memory, but in a *kintsugi* version.

> [*Kintsugi* means] golden joinery; it refers to the Japanese art of repairing broken pottery by mending the areas of breakage with lacquer dusted or mixed with powdered gold, silver or platinum. As a philosophy, it treats breakage and repair as part of the history of an object, rather than something to disguise.[3]

In my research, I call this "creative reconceptualization."[4] When you harness the power that's in your nonconscious mind, you're capable of making mental and emotional strides in your life. Through your thinking, you can actively re-create thoughts and redesign the thought interior of your mind.

I love the fact that no matter what happens, we can use our minds to change our minds. Being able to re-create is power. It means we can always do a do-over. I also love that we have such an ability to connect with others through our mind. In fact, this is a great responsibility, because we literally mirror other people's emotions and experiences if we're paying attention to them. If other people are depressed, for instance, and we focus on them, our brain will reflect their depression. And, if we spend enough time with them, there's a good chance we'll get depressed too if we don't protect our mind by deliberately and consciously choosing to process and deflect the depression.

This doesn't mean we shouldn't have empathy. In fact, our empathy increases because by noticing the effect someone's mood has on us, we are tuning in to them, and by deflecting we keep ourselves strong enough to help them—we can't help anyone if we're overwhelmed. In the same way, if we spend time with happy people, our brain reflects their expressions and actions and our mood improves!

Whatever You Think about the Most Grows

Whatever has the most energy in the nonconscious mind reflects what we've spent the most time thinking about. *Whatever we think about the most grows because we're giving it energy.* Just like a plant needs water to grow, a thought needs energy to grow.

> Whatever we think about the most grows, because we're giving it energy.

Thoughts are real things. And, like all real things, they generate energy: little packets of energy called *photons*, which are the fundamental particles of light. Albert Einstein discovered this law (photoelectric effect) and won the 1921 Nobel Prize in Physics for his work.

Though all of us have experienced photons in many ways, perhaps you've never thought of them in relation to your thoughts, so let me give you an example. You're watching someone bullying people and suddenly you find yourself almost taking a step back, and you feel disturbed. It's almost as though the person is throwing something at you. What you're experiencing is the toxic energy from that person's thoughts—and it's real.

Mental energy sucks others in. Think of hanging out with someone who's constantly depressed or negative and how you feel around them. Fear breeds fear. The fearful mind generates fearful probabilities. The depressed mind generates depressing possibilities. But the same can be said for the positive. The excited mind generates exciting possibilities. The joyful mind generates joyful possibilities. And the list goes on. We are what we think, and what we think about most will grow.

That's why we need to be discerning about who we connect with and who we listen to. We can quite literally enhance or damage each other. When we inadvertently allow others to fill our mind with their thinking, we're at their mercy. The energy from people's thoughts is real, and we need to protect ourselves from it if it's negative or grab it with both hands if it's positive. Thoughts and ideas from other people, including what we hear, read, and watch, have the potential to exert a controlling influence over our thinking, feeling, and choosing—if we let them.

However, it's interesting to note that memories formed from shared experiences will diminish within twenty-four to forty-eight hours because the proteins they're made of denature. This essentially means that they become heat energy. That's great for negative experiences, but to maintain and sustain a positive encounter, we need to focus on it for longer periods of time to maintain the benefit.

By the same token, what we're doing with our minds, our words, our attitudes, and our beliefs affects the people around us. Have you ever had anyone tell you there's a black cloud hanging over you and it's affecting them? Or that you're creating a toxic work environment by letting your stress affect everyone in the office? There's real energy being emitted from your thoughts and affecting others.

> *Dr. Leaf, I just had to tell you this: I got really angry today*
> *after being confronted with a petty trigger of mine. At*
> *first I acted on the anger but then I sat down and analyzed*
> *why I got so angry using your 5 Steps. I calmed down*
> *and was able to reconceptualize and resolve the situation*
> *before it escalated. I didn't take the anger with me!*
>
> Sandra

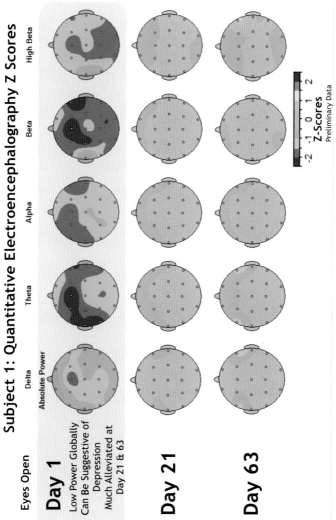

Subject 1: Quantitative Electroencephalography Z Scores

Eyes Open

Delta   Theta   Alpha   Beta   High Beta

Absolute Power

Day 1

Low Power Globally
Can Be Suggestive of
Depression
Much Alleviated at
Day 21 & 63

Day 21

Day 63

Z-Scores
-2 -1 0 1 2
Preliminary Data

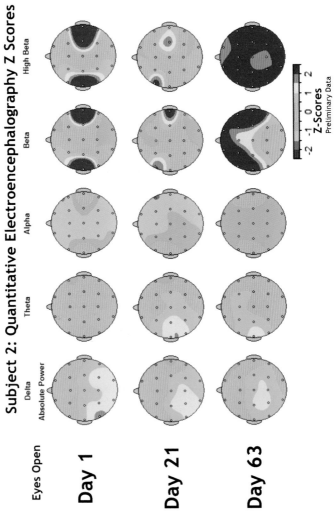

Subject 2: Quantitative Electroencephalography Z Scores

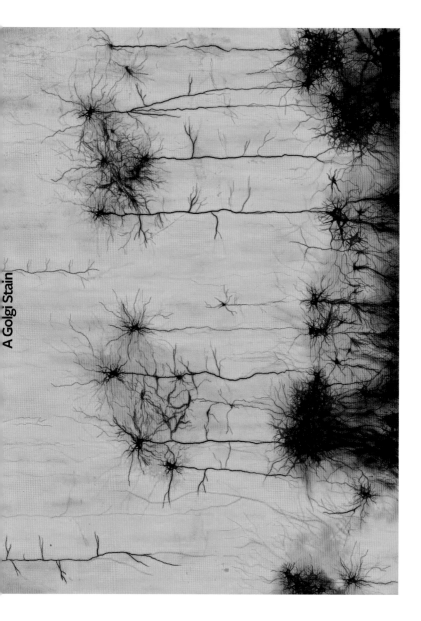

A Golgi Stain

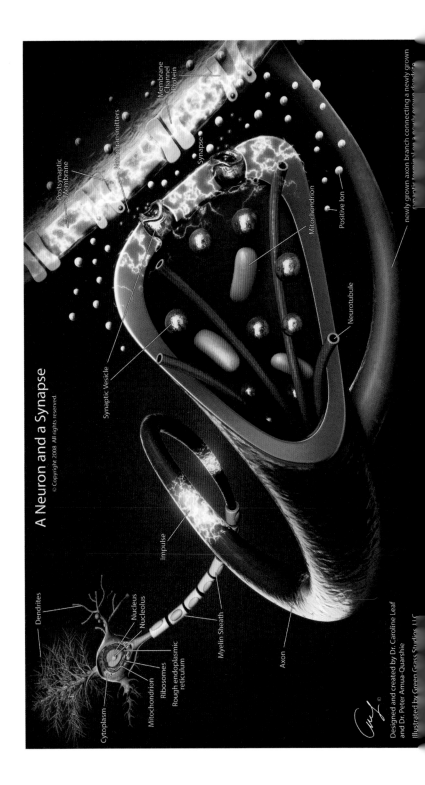

A Neuron and a Synapse

© Copyright 2008 All rights reserved.

Postsynaptic Membrane

Neurotransmitters

Membrane Channel Protein

Synapse

Mitochondrion

Positive Ion

Neurotubule

Synaptic Vesicle

newly grown axon branch connecting a newly grown
synaptic remnant on a newly grown dendrite

Impulse

Dendrites

Nucleus
Nucleolus

Cytoplasm

Mitochondrion

Ribosomes

Rough endoplasmic
reticulum

Myelin Sheath

Axon

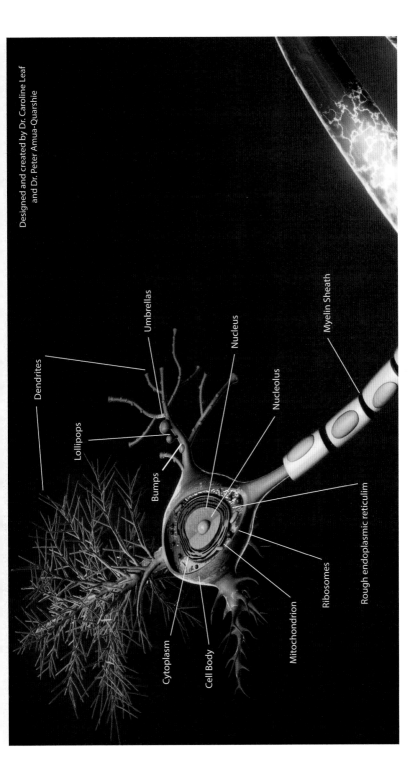

Designed and created by Dr. Caroline Leaf and Dr. Peter Amua-Quarshie

Dendrites

Umbrellas

Lollipops

Bumps

Nucleus

Nucleolus

Myelin Sheath

Cytoplasm

Cell Body

Mitochondrion

Ribosomes

Rough endoplasmic reticulim

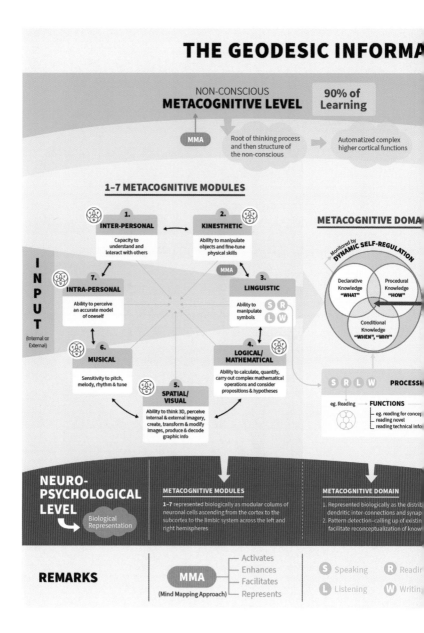

THE GEODESIC INFORMA

NON-CONSCIOUS
METACOGNITIVE LEVEL

90% of Learning

MMA → Root of thinking process and then structure of the non-conscious → Automatized complex higher cortical functions

1–7 METACOGNITIVE MODULES

1. INTER-PERSONAL
Capacity to understand and interact with others

2. KINESTHETIC
Ability to manipulate objects and fine-tune physical skills

MMA

7. INTRA-PERSONAL
Ability to perceive an accurate model of oneself

3. LINGUISTIC
Ability to manipulate symbols

S R L W

6. MUSICAL
Sensitivity to pitch, melody, rhythm & tune

5. SPATIAL/ VISUAL
Ability to think 3D, perceive internal & external imagery, create, transform & modify images, produce & decode graphic info

4. LOGICAL/ MATHEMATICAL
Ability to calculate, quantify, carry out complex mathematical operations and consider propositions & hypotheses

I N P U T
(Internal or External)

METACOGNITIVE DOMA

Monitored by **DYNAMIC SELF-REGULATION**

Declarative Knowledge "WHAT"

Procedural Knowledge "HOW"

Conditional Knowledge "WHEN", "WHY"

S R L W **PROCESS**

eg. Reading — **FUNCTIONS**
— eg. reading for concep
— reading novel
— reading technical info

NEURO-PSYCHOLOGICAL LEVEL
Biological Representation

METACOGNITIVE MODULES
1–7 represented biologically as modular colums of neuronal cells ascending from the cortex to the subcortex to the limbic system across the left and right hemispheres

METACOGNITIVE DOMAIN
1. Represented biologically as the distrib
dendritic inter-connections and synap
2. Pattern detection-calling up of existin
facilitate reconceptualization of know

REMARKS

MMA
(Mind Mapping Approach)
— Activates
— Enhances
— Facilitates
— Represents

S Speaking **R** Readir
L Listening **W** Writin

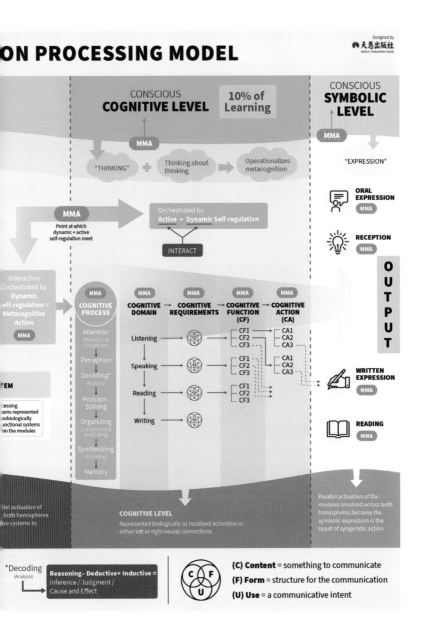

ON PROCESSING MODEL

Designed by
天恩出版社
GRACE PUBLISHING HOUSE

CONSCIOUS COGNITIVE LEVEL

10% of Learning

CONSCIOUS SYMBOLIC LEVEL

MMA

MMA

"THINKING" + Thinking about thinking → Operationalizes metacognition

"EXPRESSION"

MMA
Point at which dynamic + active self-regulation meet

Orchestrated by
Active + Dynamic Self-regulation

INTERACT

ORAL EXPRESSION
MMA

RECEPTION
MMA

Interaction
Orchestrated by
Dynamic
Self-regulation =
Metacognitive
Action

MMA

MMA
COGNITIVE PROCESS

Attention
(Allocation & Delegation)

Perception

Decoding*
(Analysis)

Problem-Solving

Organizing
(Categorizing & Associating)

Synthesizing
(Encoding)

Memory

MMA	MMA	MMA	MMA
COGNITIVE DOMAIN →	COGNITIVE REQUIREMENTS →	COGNITIVE FUNCTION (CF) →	COGNITIVE ACTION (CA)

Listening → — CF1 — CA1
 CF2 — CA2
 CF3 — CA3

Speaking → — CF1 — CA1
 CF2 — CA2
 CF3 — CA3

Reading → — CF1
 CF2
 CF3

Writing →

O U T P U T

WRITTEN EXPRESSION
MMA

READING
MMA

...TEM

...cessing
...ems represented
...robiologically
...unctional systems
...in the modules

...llel activation of
...both hemispheres
...ve systems to

COGNITIVE LEVEL
Represented biologically as localized activation in either left or right neural connections

Parallel activation of the modules involved across both hemispheres because the symbolic expression is the result of syngeristic action

*Decoding
(Analysis)
Reasoning– Deductive+ Inductive =
Inference / Judgment /
Cause and Effect

C F U

(C) Content = something to communicate
(F) Form = structure for the communication
(U) Use = a communicative intent

A Mind-Management Flow Chart

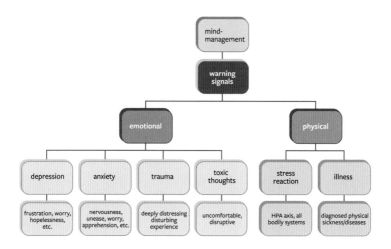

You cannot defeat darkness by running from it, nor can you conquer your inner demons by hiding them from the world. In order to defeat the darkness, you must bring it into the light.

SETH ADAM SMITH

PART TWO

THE
PRACTICAL
APPLICATION
OF THE
NEUROCYCLE

Chapter 8

The 5 Steps of the Neurocycle

In the age of technology there is constant access to vast amounts of information. The basket overflows; people get overwhelmed; the eye of the storm is not so much what goes on in the world, it is the confusion of how to think, feel, digest, and react to what goes on.

CRISS JAMI

Overview

- Mind-management, when done correctly, helps facilitate "talk" between the conscious, subconscious, and nonconscious mind.
- We are not prisoners to the contents of our mind, whether they come in the form of an anxious thought, a depressive feeling, and/or a painful memory.
- The Neurocycle builds memory effectively and in an integrated way, helping us manage the contents of our mind.
- The 5 Steps function like a delivery company, which works no matter what the parcel is, where it comes from, or where it's going. Likewise, the 5 Steps of mind-management work no matter what your issue is, where it comes from, or where it's going.

Health problems, money issues, relationship challenges, imposter syndrome, technology overload, a heavy workload, caregiving, sick family members, pandemics . . . there are so many things that can make us anxious, depressed, and stressed out. Although we've made many advances as a species, modern life is not without its own unique pressures and problems. As a result, lifestyles and life spans have been affected.

But this doesn't have to be your story. With scientific, clinically researched, and practical solutions for preventative, proactive, and strategic mind-management, I'll teach you how to foster and cultivate the power of your own thinking and direct your own brain changes. Mind-management, when done correctly, helps facilitate talk between the conscious, subconscious, and nonconscious mind. This, in turn, gets your brain waves flowing in a healthy way, optimizing brain function. You set the environment for your telomeres to grow, improving cellular aging. You learn control over the physiology of your body and the neurophysiology of your brain. And you gain control over your mental health.

> Mind-management, when done correctly, helps facilitate talk between the conscious, subconscious, and nonconscious mind.

We can learn to shape our reactions and clean up our mental mess. When we're aware of our mental power, we can catch and control intrusive thoughts that cause chaos in our minds, those ruminating, hamster-wheel thoughts that go nowhere and make us feel worse. We can learn how to really listen and tune in to how we think, feel, and choose and how others think, feel, and choose, literally designing and customizing how we react to people and events.

Really, each moment of every day needs mind-management, because each moment sets up the next, with significant mental and physical repercussions, and with your mind you can drive the brain in an organized or disorganized direction. The way you use your mind can rebuild and strengthen your brain, even when you have gone through the traumas of life. You can bring your brain under your control, no matter your past and no matter your present. You can capture and control thoughts and reconceptualize your thinking.

Jacuzzi Problems

We have a Jacuzzi bathtub, and using it is one of my favorite ways to take a mental self-care break. After a long day, a heavy workout, and a hot sauna, I love taking a long, hot bath. One night, as I was enjoying the bubbles growing around me, I realized one of the beautiful diamond earrings my children had given me for my birthday had fallen from my ear and into the water! I had to find it before it got sucked down the plug, which I had mistakenly kicked open in my panic as I realized the earring was missing. The sound of water draining didn't help calm me down. In my mind I saw the earring disappear and my having to tell my children what happened. I frantically switched off the Jacuzzi, burrowed through the bubbles to close the plug before any more water drained out, and then had to wait for the bubbles to subside before I could see if the earring had gone down the drain.

In the midst of soapy chaos and my mental mess, I got out of the tub and yelled for my husband, Mac, to come and "kill these stupid bubbles," getting terribly frustrated while I waited for a clear view. I slipped in the foam, which was now all over the bathroom floor, and hurt my knee. I ended up yelling at Mac as though this whole saga was his fault. *Why didn't he remind me to take off my earrings before bathing?*

When we finally got the foam under control, we both held our breaths while we peered into the water to find the earring. Mac saw it first and grabbed it. We both sighed in relief—me because I had found the precious gift from my children, and Mac because my tantrum was going to end and he could go back to watching the end of *Braveheart* for the thirtieth time.

I realized a number of things in this soapy saga. First, that earring could have easily been lost, as I was not immediately aware it had fallen off and had to **gather** the relevant information. Second, **reflecting** back, my panicky feelings were a normal reaction under the circumstances—the root of the panic was my fear of losing something special. To solve the problem, I had to have a plan, something to do—I needed clear, logical steps. I then went into a kind of **write** mode in my head, creating a plan of action that moved me forward and out of my frozen fear mode. As I did this, I had to **recheck** that my plan would work, because it was taking more time and effort than expected to pat down that mountain of bubbles on my own. I decided to **actively reach** out to my husband for help (even though I got a bit frustrated at first!).

So, as I was looking for my lost earring, I went through 5 Steps:

1. Gather
2. Reflect
3. Write
4. Recheck
5. Active Reach

This is a ridiculous example, I know. But it's a helpful way to understand how the 5 Steps work. *They* are definitely not silly, and I share this simple story to show you how our neuroplasticity can be self-directed.

We are not prisoners to the contents of our mind, whether they come in the form of an anxious thought, a depressive feeling, or a painful memory. Mind-management sets us free. Though these 5 Steps take some time and effort, at their core they're simple and rewarding and can be mastered over time. In fact, the more you use them, the easier they are and the more adaptable you become at managing your mind and lifestyle.

Most of us know the basics of living a good lifestyle. We need to have good habits like connecting with others in deep and meaningful ways, eating real food mindfully, exercising regularly, and managing stress to be healthy. So, where do the 5 Steps fit into a good lifestyle? Well, as I'm sure you know, it's one thing to know what to do, and another thing entirely to do it. The 5 Steps are, at their core, a *delivery system*. They deliver the parcel of knowledge to your brain and body so you can go from knowing how good something is for you to actually living a good life. What this means is that you can learn to use your mind to discipline your mind (your thinking, feeling, and choosing) and go from *knowing* about good lifestyle decisions to actually *making* good lifestyle decisions.

The Neurocycle provides a way of *accessing and directing the mind behind the mindset*. This means that we can learn to control the mind behind our daily struggles, the things that blindside us, our traumas, the meal, the exercise plan, and so on. If your mind is not right, nothing else will be right because your mind is behind everything you do. Remember: you can't even go three seconds without thinking!

The Foundational Principles of the Neurocycle

As I've mentioned before, the 5 Steps are kind of like doing your own brain surgery. As you direct your mind-in-action, you change your brain and mental space for the better, getting rid of toxic thoughts and building good, healthy thoughts and habits.

The foundational principles of this mind-management tool, the Neurocycle, are embracing, processing, and reconceptualizing, and the 5 Steps are your "surgical instruments" for doing so.

- Step 1 (Gather) involves **embracing** the toxic thought, habit, or trauma (*cutting open with the scalpel*).
- Steps 2 and 3 (Reflect and Write) are the **processing** steps (*performing the surgery*).

- Steps 4 and 5 (Recheck and Active Reach) are the **reconceptualizing** steps (*closing up and healing*).

Embracing means acknowledging, facing, accepting, and willingly and mindfully gathering awareness of the emotional and physical warning signals your brain and body send you.

Processing is the "mental autopsy" part of the mental surgery. It entails deep, intentional, and focused thinking, which forces the conscious mind and nonconscious mind to connect.

Reconceptualizing means redesigning the thinking, feeling, and choosing behind the thought by learning from the lessons of the past. When you reconceptualize a thought, you're examining the information, emotions, and choices that led to that thought. In doing this, you're looking at what happened or what you were thinking from a new angle, another perspective that makes it manageable, so that you no longer feel crippled by pain—the level of your emotional distress changes.

Reconceptualization helps you build a replacement thought that has the lessons from the toxic thought as its foundation. It literally redesigns your thinking and your brain, enabling you to progress forward. I'm sure you have already experienced this many times in your life, you just may not have known the actual steps or science behind it. Think of a time you went through something very challenging, got through to the other side, and then, almost instinctively, felt the need to share your story to help others because your own reconceptualization process was so life-transforming.

When I think of reconceptualization I often think of a young woman I met who had lost her husband in a hurricane; she witnessed as his head was severed from his body by flying debris. This is an unimaginable trauma, the kind you never really get over. However, in the midst of her grief and pain, she chose to reconceptualize her pain and grief by accepting she would never get over it because it was terrible, but she knew she had to find a way to make it mean something in order to cope. She did this by pouring her energy into helping others process their grief.

Reconceptualization can apply to serious traumas like this, as well as everyday life struggles. Here is an example of something that is not as extreme. My husband, Mac, and I work together, so this means we're together 24/7. I've had to self-regulate and use the 5 Steps to go through the process of reconceptualizing when it comes to meetings, because he has a way of interrupting. I used to get really irritated and snappy, but I've reconceptualized this from *He's not listening and keeps interrupting* to *Let me really listen to what he's asking and hear the deeper meaning, and ask him kindly not to interrupt.* I altered how I saw what he was doing by listening to him differently, and it's changed everything about our discussions for the better. Mac's very considerate now about letting me finish my train of thought before he asks questions. And I answer him patiently and with kindness. It's a little shift that's had great rewards. But it took me a full sixty-three days of using the Neurocycle to really make it work. Now it's a habit.

Throughout this book are testimonies of people whose lives have changed in different ways from using the 5 Steps. Read them to encourage yourself, especially when times get hard. Like them, you will get to the other side of the pain! In fact, whenever you get some good advice or tips from a friend, counselor, or loved one, slot them into the 5 Steps so that you can learn how to use them in your life and not just read them and say, "Oh, that's amazing! I must do that." I do this all the time!

Embracing, Processing, and Reconceptualizing

So, as you use step 1, Gather, you **embrace** the feeling of anxiety or depression as an emotional warning signal that something is going on. You also tune in to the physical warning signal of your stress, such as an increased heartrate or a headache or stomachache. You embrace the information attached to the emotions. You do this in a celebratory way, not because you're celebrating the painful memories but because now you're conscious of them, which means you can change them. The celebration is in the changing!

Embracing is one of the hardest tasks, because it requires us to admit we're struggling and face the issue, thought, or feeling head-on. Our ego is challenged, and our sense of comfort and security is threatened. It's at this point that many people run in the opposite direction, either out of fear or because of guilt or shame due to the incorrect practice of making emotions a part of their identity. However, it's this very awareness that instructs the body to release specific chemicals and switch genes on and off, directing the best flow of different energy frequencies of the brain. It even increases blood flow and oxygen to the front of the brain, helping repair the damage from the emotional intensity of trauma and chronic unmanaged stress. Here are some simple tips to make the embracing a little more palatable.

1. Acknowledge that emotions, thoughts, trauma, and past experiences are not your identity. For example, you're challenging the *feelings* of shame, not saying you *are* shame.

2. Accept that pain is a nonnegotiable when doing the work to heal. Tell yourself that it will end eventually, even if it doesn't feel like it will in the moment.

3. Always remember that you're never alone in this journey and that you deserve the love and support your loved ones give you as you reach out and ask for help.

4. Remind yourself of past tough experiences you have overcome despite fear or uncertainty.

5. Keep in mind that this painful part won't last forever, and the sooner you learn to embrace it, the sooner you will move through it.

6. And most exciting of all—as soon as you embrace it, the thought has weakened and is in the process of

change—even if it doesn't feel like it. Our nervous system and nonconscious change before we're conscious of this change and experiencing it in our life.

Not embracing your feelings doesn't make them go away. If they don't come out, they'll go into your body, cells, DNA, and mind and will explode in volcanic mode at some point—there's absolutely no getting away from this. Denying the existence of the emotions or thoughts is a defense mechanism that may help you avoid discomfort for a short period of time, but it doesn't promote healing and will ultimately take you to a breaking point.

After embracing, you move into the **processing** stage, which are steps 2 and 3, Reflect and Write. This involves deep reflection using the classic "w" questions—who, what, when, where, why, and how. Writing these thoughts down plays a massive role in organizing your thinking in order to identify the perspective and find the root: the origin of the thinking, feeling, and choosing behind them. These deep reflection and writing steps are good places to use a lot of the directed neuroplasticity techniques we'll talk about in chapter 9.

The processing stage is also hard emotional work, especially when dealing with trauma, so be careful not to compare your processing to someone else's or put a time frame on it. For example, you may need a few rounds of 63-day cycles to resolve those deep mental scars you've been avoiding for a while. Don't assume that you must deal with these issues within one 63-day cycle or whatever time limit you impose on yourself, as this will set you up for failure.

After processing, you then **reconceptualize** this thought, which is step 4, Recheck, and step 5, Active Reach. You do this by evaluating what you've written, which is a way of looking at your behaviors and communication: how they've impacted your life, where they come from, and what other ways you can perceive them so their impact on your life is neutralized.

It's important to remember that *you* control this process. In fact, you direct it, because this is your life experience. Use the directed neuroplasticity techniques here as well to make this process easier. The goal of reconceptualization is to illuminate the change and honor the process of being human and going through life. It is *not* a Band-Aid on a deep wound, it's not like the process of tattoo removal, it's not the creation of a competing "correct" thought that if you think of it often enough will take precedence over the toxic thought. Reconceptualization is the recognition and removal of the chains that bind you to the past—it's the trial becoming the testimony. It's incorporating your story, which is now redesigned (with the pain accepted and neutralized); it's not ignoring or suppressing what you've gone through but rather honoring the past for the growth it has brought into your life and incorporating this change into your day-to-day living. It switches your flaws, mistakes, and pain into your secret weapon—something valuable you've learned from, for growth and for learning to love your history.

The Japanese have a brilliant concept that really captures what reconceptualizing is, called *kintsugi*, which I mentioned earlier. This is the art of repairing broken pottery with lacquer that has been dusted or mixed with gold, silver, or platinum powder. A broken ceramic vase is repaired rather than discarded, and is turned into something uniquely beautiful—the breaks are gilded into amazing patterns that highlight them instead of hide them.

A therapist, pastor, counselor, or coach cannot know what's best for you, although they can help you figure it out for yourself. But only you truly know your own experience. You're the expert on your life. The most effective way to utilize something like therapy is to see it as a way to problem-solve with a partner—to put the gilding into the breaks of the ceramic vase together, which is what I did with my patients in my twenty-five years of clinical practice. However, now you can use the 5 Steps, which is how *you* manage your mind all day long. It's what you do in between therapy, coaching, or talking to a friend or loved one and how you can get through the day.

The best way to get the most out of your mind is to use the Neurocycle daily. In my clinical practice and clinical trials, the subjects that **rigorously and consistently applied these 5 Steps over the 63-day periods** benefited the most in terms of reducing their anxiety and depression, learning issues, and so on, which helped them feel like they were more equipped to face challenges and deal with their issues.

Going Deeper into the 5 Steps of the Neurocycle

The Neurocycle is a scientific five-step process that helps you use your mind and brain in a way that directs the neuroplasticity of your brain to your benefit, and in doing so, improves your mind, brain, and body health.

These 5 Steps drive neuroplasticity in the brain. They're the steps the mind goes through, as it builds thoughts and detoxes thoughts, which change the structure of the brain. So, they're the science of thought put into a very simplified process. Each of these steps is based on neuroscientific research on how we build thoughts and memories, which are real things, into the brain. Going through the steps sequentially is a process I call *neurocycling*.

When should you use this? All the time, because you're always using your mind! You don't even go three seconds without thinking; the Neurocycle helps you master this mind-in-action and become the boss of your brain. It is a way to harness your thinking power.

The easiest way to understand the 5 Steps is to look back at the thought tree in chapter 7 alongside the image below. Look at it from the branches to the tree trunk to the roots. Step 1 is gathering awareness of the branches and leaves, which are your behaviors and their attached emotions. Step 2 is focusing on the whole tree to try to make sense of it—the branches, trunk, and roots, or the detail of your behaviors and emotions, what perspective they bring, and where they come from.

Step 3 is writing, which is a revealing process of bringing the memories of the thoughts out into the open and into your conscious mind. Step 4 is a pruning and grafting process based on the discoveries you make in steps 1 and 2, like the kintsugi process discussed earlier. Step 5 is a stabilizing and consolidating process, where you allow the new plant to settle a little before you do more work on it, and where you wait for the cracks to dry before adding more gold lacquer.

Now, let's look at these 5 Steps in a little more detail. The first step is to **Gather**. This means choosing to pay attention to your behaviors (what you say and do) and increasing your conscious

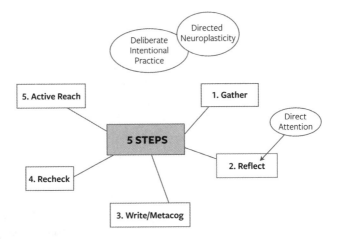

awareness. This awareness becomes a directing force that instructs the brain how to respond on a chemical, energy, and genetic level. You're literally pulling the thought tree into the conscious mind to deal with it by gathering awareness of it. You can change something only when you're conscious of it—that's why the nonconscious tries to catch your attention by sending you emotional and physical warning signals through the subconscious mind. Never ignore these prompts, no matter how much they may upset you or someone else. They're rich with information.

With the Gather step, you embrace the physical, emotional, and informational memories intertwined within your thoughts—you start "pulling up" the branches, leaves, tree trunk, and roots.

This step forces you to really tune in to the prompts from your nonconscious mind. The goal is to choose to pay attention and focus on your behaviors in terms of the signals coming from your nonconscious mind. Questions to ask at this step could be:

1. What are you experiencing through your five senses? Gather awareness of these physical warning signals emerging from your body.
2. What is the information in the thoughts bubbling up from your nonconscious mind into your conscious mind right at this moment? Gather awareness of this information, noting how many thoughts there are and what they are.
3. What feelings are attached to the information the thought contains? Every thought has emotions as part of its structure—they're stored in the nonconscious mind. When thoughts move into the conscious mind, we feel the emotions of them. Just gather awareness of the feelings attached to each thought.

The second step of the Neurocycle is to **Reflect**. This is where you *ask*, *answer*, and *discuss* what you have gathered awareness of in step 1 through the "w" questions. The purpose of this step is to understand your behaviors and communication, and how they're related to what you're thinking, feeling, choosing, and experiencing to find the origin, or the root cause, of what you're experiencing.

The aim of this step is to shift your focus from the behaviors to the thought that triggered these behaviors, then to the perspective, then to the root cause. This challenges the brain to move into a higher gear, which is what it's designed for: deep, intellectual thinking. This reflective step makes a thought susceptible to change by activating the theta, delta, and gamma waves in waves of energy and weakening its connections in your mind. As your insight into what's going on grows, you can start directing the energy flow in the brain that tells the brain and body which chemicals should be released, which genes should be activated and deactivated, where chemicals should flow to, and, ultimately, what neuroplastic structural and chemical and energy changes should occur in the brain.

Another way to do the Reflect step is to use the "5 Why" technique created by Sakichi Toyoda, the Japanese industrialist, inventor, and founder of Toyota Industries. The method is simple: you just ask yourself *Why?* five times as a way of drilling down to the root issue. However, if you feel the need to use all of the "w" questions more than five times, you can—whatever works for you.

Additionally, in this step you question the thought or emotion by asking yourself, *Is this based on a fact or assumption? Is what I am thinking true or false?* Too often we cause ourselves more mental distress than necessary because we don't stop to question our thoughts. This questioning really loosens up thoughts in the brain, making it easier to reconceptualize. Some more questions to guide you at this step include:

1. What am I experiencing physically as I reflect on the thought? Try to describe this in as much detail as possible.
2. What is the information on the thought? Try to describe in as much detail as possible by answering the "w" questions: who, what, when, where, why, and how.
3. What feelings are attached to the information in the thought? Try to describe in as much detail and as specifically as possible.

Step 3 is to **Write**. The brain makes or "writes" proteins when genes are switched on by your thinking, feeling, and choosing. When you write down what you've been thinking about in step 2, it consolidates memory and adds clarity to what you're thinking about, allowing you to better see the area that needs to be detoxed or the thought that needs to be built. It essentially allows you to visualize your thoughts, bringing suppressed thoughts out of the nonconscious to be reconceptualized.

Writing brings order out of chaos by "putting your brain on paper." If we don't get our suppressed thoughts out, they stay rooted in our mind, causing mental and physical damage. Toxic thoughts have incorrectly folded proteins and an imbalanced electromagnetic and chemical flow with less oxygen and blood flow. They're unhealthy and can lead to inflammation in the brain, which can cause all sorts of issues.

Research shows that writing can even improve immune system function![1] We saw this in our clinical trials with the experimental group, who were using all 5 Steps. When they went through step 3, they experienced a statistically significant drop in their cortisol and homocysteine levels, which predict immune system health. When you write, you stimulate a flow of neurotransmitters in your brain that help clear your thinking. You activate an area in your brain called the basal ganglia, which allows for cognitive fluency. This improves the smoothness and insightfulness of your reasoning, and you can start seeing and understanding things you didn't before. Writing can be done on paper, on your phone, or even as recorded voice memos. Writing can also be done using a process I developed called a Metacog, which is an incredibly effective way of getting into the nonconscious mind and finding the root issue. See appendix B for how to make a Metacog.

Step 4 is to **Recheck** what you've written. This is an *editing process* (pruning and grafting the tree) to check for accuracy and to find patterns in your thinking, kind of like a mental autopsy. You shift from the "why, what" to more of the "how, when" questions. This process allows you to reconceptualize the toxic thought and turn it into a new, healthy thought habit in the spirit of the *kintsugi* philosophy. In this step, you'll evaluate what you've written in step 3 and think about the new healthy thought you want to build. You will also be able to rethink your reaction to the information, evaluating how the toxic thought you're working on is changing, and then reconceptualizing it—little by little, day by day.

Some questions to guide you as you do this step include:

1. What am I experiencing physically? Is there a pattern? How is this linked to the information and feelings of the thought?
2. What are the patterns of the information in my thoughts? How can I reconceptualize this information?
3. What feelings are attached to the information in the thought? What patterns do I see? How can I reconceptualize these feelings?

Step 5 is what I call **Active Reach**. This is where you *practice*, *apply*, and *teach* what you've been working on. An Active Reach is the action you do during the day to practice the reconceptualized thought, and it comes from the Recheck step. You decide what the action is each day as you work through the 5 Steps. It's meant to be simple, quick, efficient, and easy to apply. It could be a breathing exercise or a simple statement you say to remind yourself what you learned from the first four steps during that particular day. It can be as simple as "practice not saying *if only* today."

You can do the same Active Reach as the previous day or a brand-new Active Reach; that's completely up to you. The Active Reach step is essential; change requires action, not just information. Application is essential to growth—it's practice, and practice makes perfect.

Some questions to guide you as you do this step include:

1. What is my physical trigger?
2. What is my reconceptualized information?
3. What are my reconceptualized feelings?

Now, create an Active Reach with your answers. For example, "When I experience the physical trigger of _____ I will tell myself _____ and choose to feel _____."

Let's finish this section by looking at all this information in a different form: a table of the 5 Steps of the Neurocycle and the corresponding brain, body, and mind responses.

TABLE 4. The 5 Steps of The Neurocycle

Step	Definition	Brain Response	Body Response (Physical Signals)	Mind Response (Emotional and Informational Signals)
1. Gather the physical, emotional, and informational warning signals.	Becoming aware of all the physical, informational, and emotional warning signals that are coming into your mind from the external environment through the five senses and understanding the internal environment of your mind. This self-regulating awareness is how you train yourself to become aware of the information in the thought.	Increased alpha bridge and increased activity in amygdala and hippocampus. The circuits and columns around the basal ganglia (deep inside the middle of the brain) get the brain into a state of expectation, preparing it to build the new, incoming information.	Increase in HPA axis activity; changes in neuroendocrine, immune, and cardiovascular systems. Experienced as an adrenaline rush, heart palpitations, tightening of muscles, tongue stuck to the roof of the mouth, headaches, GI symptoms, and so on.	The nonconscious mind sends prompts through the subconscious mind to the conscious mind in the form of physical, informational, and emotional warning signals—these are experienced as a hovering awareness, anxiety, angst, or a tip-of-the-tongue, just-aware sense of discomfort.
2. Reflect on the physical, emotional, and informational warning signals.	Thinking deeply to understand and going beyond storing facts and answers to storing key reconceptualized concepts and strategic thoughts. When you reflect, you specifically focus on one thought's information,	Increased beta and burst of high beta and gamma waves of energy, predominantly in the center and front of the brain, which happens when we focus our thinking. There will also be an increase in alpha and theta energy as	Heightened activity in the HPA axis, the stress response.	Conscious and nonconscious mind are working very closely together as you do the mental autopsy on the thought, dissecting its emotions, information, and physical impact, and the deeper you think, the more effectively this happens.

Step	Definition	Brain Response	Body Response (Physical Signals)	Mind Response (Emotional and Informational Signals)
*You can do steps 2 and 3 simultaneously or separately.	emotions, and physical warning signals. It is a directed and deep, self-regulated intellectual process and a disciplined way of thinking that has the elements of attention regulation, controlling ragging, and preventing chaotic thoughts from moving uncontrolled through the mind.	the nonconscious and conscious mind are stimulated to work together to drag up the nonconscious activity—the thoughts driving you. Neuroplasticity is dominant because, as you consciously and deliberately focus your thinking, you start redesigning your brain structure.		
3. **Write**	Writing on paper (or on your phone/computer) starts to bring clarity because you are literally emptying your brain on paper. A flow of neurotransmitters in your brain begins that actually helps clear your thinking. You activate the basal ganglia of the brain, which allows for cognitive fluency, or clear thinking.	Increase in the alpha bridge so there can be insightful connection between the conscious and nonconscious mind.	The action of writing allows a lot of transferring of anxious energy from the body and brain to your pen.	Writing increases feelings of autonomy and clarity, and the effect is cumulative—each day you will get more and more clarity and order to help clean the mental mess.

Step	Definition	Brain Response	Body Response (Physical Signals)	Mind Response (Emotional and Informational Signals)
4. Recheck the physical, emotional, and informational warning signals.	A revealing, exciting process and a progressive "moving forward" step: revisiting where you are and looking at how to make change happen, you wire in what changes you want. You get to design your new healthy thought to replace the toxic thought. You're seeing in a different way the toxic thoughts that create such powerful internal conflicts in your mind and are capable of causing radical electrochemical imbalances. In rechecking, you are not only looking at how you go about dealing with your circumstances but are also thinking through your reactions again, evaluating the toxicity levels, and retranscribing them.	Serious "brain surgery" that optimizes all the energy frequencies of the brain. It specifically activates theta, a healing wave. Completing the first three steps will have stimulated major neuroplastic activity, putting your brain in a highly active and dynamic state of change. This is the perfect state to be in to rewire. By consciously becoming aware of your thought life, you are retranscribing, reconceptualizing, and changing your underlying neuronal networks.	A positive, looking-for-the-solution step. It feels safe because you are balancing the nervous system and brain and making stress work for you and not against you.	When thoughts are activated and pushed into the conscious mind, they enter a labile state—meaning they can be altered. When a memory is in this plastic state, it can be modified, toned down, or retranscribed and reconceptualized by interfering with protein synthesis—an important molecular process in thought building.

Step	Definition	Brain Response	Body Response (Physical Signals)	Mind Response (Emotional and Informational Signals)
	While Gather, Reflect, and Write are hugely instrumental in this process, Recheck is a self-reflective process that has the purpose of getting free from internal conflicts with positive planning of the way out. It is a constructive and cumulative step that takes you through the problem.			
5. Active Reach	Practicing your newly re-conceptualized thoughts and getting into the mode of rehearsing things mentally, which is a great everyday part of mind-management. Each time you do this, you change the strength of the memory by adding energy,	The "doing" nature of Active Reach results in ungluing the branches from your thought trees and rewiring new ones. There will be a lot of beta and gamma as you build new networks and as this learning is taking place. Steps 1 to 4 have loosened and weakened the	Neurochemicals flow such as oxytocin, which remolds, dopamine, which increases motivation and focus, and serotonin, which makes you feel good. These chemicals also weaken the toxic branches. The "glue" starts moving away from the toxic tree toward the	The conscious mind is very actively working with the nonconscious mind to design the new thought trees.

Step	Definition	Brain Response	Body Response (Physical Signals)	Mind Response (Emotional and Informational Signals)
	and the more energy, the more impact the memory will have in your life in terms of your communication and behavior.	branches, but step 5 literally destroys them. Here's how: the dendritic branches, with all the information and emotions, are attached to a cell body with a glue-like protein—like branches grafted to a tree trunk. There is more "glue" on the branches that are used the most, so when you shift your attention from the negative, toxic thought to the positive, healthy, new replacement thought, three things happen. The electromagnetic and quantum signals from your decision to change (1) attack the branches of the toxic thoughts, (2) weaken them, and (3) transfer the energy to the new thought, because healthy signals are more powerful than negative thoughts.	healthy reconceptualized thought "tree."	

I love all of your analogies, like the waves in the sea making wakes and how that is likened to our experience of trauma. All of this has helped me to understand that I was a victim and it is okay—that for many years I really struggled with suicidal thoughts and very low self-worth. I also had a lot of pain from my upbringing. When I had this vision, it helped heal me deeply and restore me. My core was healed. Thank you from the bottom of my heart.

ABI

Chapter 9

Directing Your Brain for Change

Overview

- We have within us the ability to tap into a state of self-awareness that allows us to develop a sense of peaceful control, a mental space necessary for coping and overcoming.

- Essentially, when you use your ability to stand outside of yourself and observe your own thinking (the MPA), your senses can tune in to the detail of the "now moment"—an enriching experience that will help you feel happier and more at peace.

- The discomfort zones are the physical, emotional, and informational warning signals from physical, emotional, and informational memories in a thought. These warning signals are invitations to look inward. If you cannot sit with them and listen to them, you run the risk of losing the opportunity to gain priceless information that will help with your healing.

- Not only can we rewire our brain but we can regenerate it as well! Changing our mind and brain is also much easier to do and more common than we think—in fact, our brain is always changing, and we drive the direction of change.

To get the optimal energy balance in the brain, which facilitates optimal blood and oxygen flow as well, you can use some specific and focused practices to help you think through things more clearly as you work through the 5 Steps.

Directed Neuroplasticity Practices

These directed neuroplasticity practices activate the alpha bridge, connecting our conscious mind with our nonconscious mind, which is key in mind-management.

1. Self-Regulation

The overarching goal of neurocycling for mind-management is to develop your self-regulation. Self-regulation develops the more you use it. This isn't a practice to be used on occasion. It's the overarching philosophy behind the 5 Steps. Our minds are by nature self-regulatory, because we are able to self-regulate every ten seconds. Our neuroplastic brains need and thrive on self-regulation.

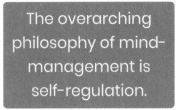

The overarching philosophy of mind-management is self-regulation.

By definition, self-regulation is the conscious awareness and regulation of:

> what and how you are thinking, feeling, and choosing at any one moment in time;
>
> your long-term established thoughts with their embedded physical, emotional, and informational memories; and
>
> your communication with others (what you say and do) and how it impacts both yourself and others.

Whatever we say and do is first a thought. This thought is a real thing that occupies mental real estate. By the same token, looking at what we say and do will lead us to the thought, which, in turn, leads us to the mind-in-action behind that thought. *Self-regulation is being aware of this process and adjusting it as necessary.*

For example, let's say you constantly say or think negative things about yourself—self-regulation of this behavior involves noticing the impact of your thoughts, words, and tone on yourself, and asking yourself why you do this in the first place. This helps you figure out the thought behind your behavior.

The self-regulation that happens on the conscious level is called *active self-regulation*, while that which happens on the nonconscious level is *dynamic self-regulation*. Active self-regulation happens only when we're awake; dynamic self-regulation is going on 24/7. When we quiet our minds through daydreaming, reading, and thinking deeply, we're allowing active (conscious mind) and dynamic (nonconscious mind) self-regulation to work together, which brings balance and coherence in the brain.

Here's how this works: about ten seconds before you're fully consciously aware of the thought and possible ways of responding to that thought, your nonconscious mind is working incredibly quickly and intelligently, at about a million operations per second, to sort out any imbalances and disequilibrium. This is dynamic self-regulation. General nonconscious activity goes on 24/7 at 10^{27} operations per second. Your nonconscious mind is literally using your brain, scanning it at quantum speeds to find all associated thoughts with their intertwined memories and belief systems, in order to help you react in the best way. This is an integrated, associative, and creative process with the purpose of guiding you to make the right decisions.

Then, at around half a second before you're fully aware, the subconscious mind starts prompting you. Remember, we have conscious bursts of activity around forty times a second.

The exciting thing is that we can train ourselves to be increasingly self-aware and self-regulated to the point that we *tune in to* these bursts around every ten seconds, or approximately six times a minute. With training, you can teach yourself to self-regulate the thoughts popping into your mind all the time while you're awake: this is living in a state of conscious awareness. This is quite a challenge but something you can train yourself to do using the 5 Steps.

Hypervigilance

It's important to note, however, that the vigilance associated with the process of self-regulation can shift into hypervigilance—what we do when we go into "watchman mode" and look for threats. Of course, we have periods in our life where we need to be hypervigilant to survive, but we can't live on edge like that all the time.

We also don't want to shift into a *hypo*vigilant state, where we suppress too much or become too reactive. These both happen when we don't apply mind-management appropriately to our situation. Below are some signs you are becoming hyper- or hypo-vigilant. Knowing certain signs will help you catch yourself before it's too late.

Signs of hypervigilance:

- Having a hovering feeling of anxiety
- Being unable to relax even when doing relaxing things
- Battling to daydream or just think
- Watching people closely, looking for signs they will do or say something wrong
- Feeling a constant sense of unease
- Being very jumpy
- Distrusting everyone
- Always seeing the negative in people and situations and not being able to accept or enjoy when good things happen

- Fighting to focus in conversations
- Avoiding facing issues by using distractions
- Having nightmares and vivid dreams that feel very real

Signs of hypovigilance:

- Suppressing feelings often and for long periods of time, then overreacting and exploding at a seemingly tiny trigger
- Having no filters in conversation
- Failing to notice the impact of words and actions on others
- Failing to learn from mistakes

We can maintain a healthy level of vigilance as we use the Neurocycle. There's no quick fix, because we will have to keep practicing the 5 Steps to make this self-regulated behavior a habit.

Peaceful Control

We have within us the ability to tap into a state of self-awareness that allows us to develop a sense of peaceful control despite whatever is going on around us, a mental space that is necessary for coping and overcoming. That's when our active self-regulation works with our dynamic self-regulation. It's the space where you can cry, express your emotions, and even freak out if you need to—you're processing what is going on but are still in a self-regulated state, which means you have a feeling of peace even when things may be unresolved.

The Neurocycle helps us achieve this state by giving us a way of catching and controlling those messy thoughts that cause chaos and mental mess. We *can learn* how to really listen and tune in to ourselves and others, literally designing and customizing how we react.

2. The 30–90 Second Rule—the "Regret Zone"

The 30–90 Second Rule is a directed neuroplasticity practice you can use any time you need to. As you experience something, whether it's an event, circumstance, spoken word, or something else, for the first few seconds, your brain and nonconscious mind are dynamically self-regulating this incoming information. They're adjusting to and organizing it in terms of your energy levels and physiology.[1] This initial biochemical and electrical surge of any given thought or feeling lasts anywhere from thirty to ninety seconds, which is an adjustment period and not the best time to respond to what you're experiencing.

Generally, this is the space where we react impulsively and say and do things we wish we hadn't—the "regret zone," I like to call it. I'm sure you, like me, have done this countless times. And if you decide to act on the mental mess you created by reacting in those first seconds, things can quickly spiral out of control. If you keep staying there, long after the thirty to ninety seconds has passed, this is a choice that can become a bad habit.

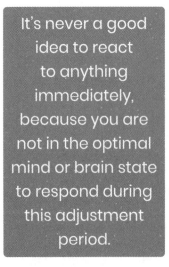

It's never a good idea to react to anything immediately, because you are not in the optimal mind or brain state to respond during this adjustment period.

It's never a good idea to react to anything immediately, because you're not in the optimal mind or brain state to respond during this adjustment period. If you do react too quickly, which can and will happen, try not to allow your toxic emotions to last longer than ninety seconds. In order to feel an emotion, we need to think about a thought in which the emotional memories are stored, which then stimulates an emotional circuit in our brain. This, in turn, creates a physiological response in our bodies. If it's a toxic, stressful, or acute situation, waiting these few seconds is invaluable. It will help the multitude of neurochemical and physiological responses to settle enough to enable you to think, feel, and choose with more order and less chaos.

Knowing what the regret zone is and using it as a "catch that thought" tool will allow you to manage your reactions. We'll save ourselves a lot of angst, as well as relationship issues, by avoiding toxic, impulsive responses that exacerbate a situation.

The goal of this 30–90 Second Rule is to help you get into a sharp, clear, and focused state of mind, one that is open to options, possibilities, and solutions. Here are a few things you can do in those seconds:

1. Do some deep belly breathing—at least ten rounds.
2. Go into a different room and just yell at the top of your lungs or as loud as you can for as long as you can.
3. Do something physical like a few sprints, jumping jacks, burpees, anything to channel the stress and intense emotions.
4. If you can't do any of the above, imagine the person in front of you shrinking down to ant size.

Remember, even if a thought or emotion feels urgent and is demanding a response from you, you are the boss. You don't need to respond to every emotion, word, or action.

As mentioned already, this is a directed neuroplasticity practice you can use to get the optimal energy balance in the brain, which will help you think through things more clearly as you work through the 5 Steps.

3. The Quantum Zeno Effect (QZE)

Although it sounds really strange, the QZE is one of my favorite directed neuroplasticity practices for mind-management. Essentially, it's based on the principle that deliberate, intentional, conscious, and repeated effort allows learning to take place. It's kind of like a mental and physical rehearsal that induces changes in the brain. We do this all day long, because we're always building thoughts into our neuroplastic brain in response to everything that's going on around us, so we may as well direct the process!

Whatever you think about the most will grow. You're either building chaos into your brain and making a mental mess, which can cause brain damage, or you're building order into your brain and cleaning up the mental mess, boosting your brain health. The overarching principle of the QZE is that whatever you pay attention to will get energy and therefore grow in your mind and brain, like watering a plant, so it's very important to train yourself to QZE in the right direction! Progressive change is based on positive, incremental progress—a tiny bit at a time. After a few weeks of these kinds of little changes, your brain will alter substantively, and if you keep this up for months you can literally build a brain that is habituated to operate in a certain way. This is what the 63-day Neurocycle can help you achieve: top-notch neuroplasticity based on self-regulated, healthy decisions.

> Whatever you think about the most will grow.

An easy and helpful way to apply the QZE is to *really* focus on the positive to the negative, in a 3:1 ratio.[2] This means that for every negative thought or feeling that comes to mind, counter it with three positive thoughts. This will help to maintain a balance in energy (quantum) waves in the brain so you can think clearly, build resilience, and rewire healthy thought trees.

Why a 3:1 ratio? Research by Dr. Barbara Frederickson has shown that there's a tipping point of at least this ratio of positivity to negativity to keep the brain in balance.[3] Toxic emotional states can cause too much high beta and high gamma energy, which make us feel awful and cause the energy in the brain to swish violently about like a tsunami, which we see as red spots, or foci, on the head maps of the qEEG. In order to rebalance this energy, the nonconscious mind grabs our attention through emotional and physical warning signals to tell us to fix it, and the fix requires managing what we focus on and think—the QZE.

Every time you have a negative thought, use it as a prompt to think of three positive things you have in your life, such as three things you're proud of yourself for, three things you're grateful for, three things that make you smile, three things that are beautiful—whatever works for you. You are essentially using the negative thought as a habit loop trigger to help you recognize what to change, but you are "padding" the negative with the positive, which is healthier for the brain.

One important distinction I want you to remember is that a negative thought isn't necessarily a toxic thought. Sometimes thinking about the worst-case scenario for a limited time period can help us not only prepare for anything so we're not blindsided but also give our minds the opportunity to be creative and imagine solutions—and to be realistic. The two important keys to preventing negative thoughts from becoming toxic thoughts are:

1. Follow up all negative thoughts with three positive thoughts to avoid ruminating and spiraling into a cycle of negativity.

2. Set a time limit on how long you spend focusing on the negative. Under five minutes is what I would recommend.

4. The Multiple Perspective Advantage (MPA)

A directed neuroplasticity practice that can help us calm down, especially in heavy emotional and tough-to-face situations, is the MPA. When you are processing a toxic emotion, you can feel "under the weather" and shape your thoughts by your negativity. We need to remember that thoughts can become distorted if we lose the joy of the *now* moment. Negativity or toxicity creates those blocks of "tsunami" energy in the brain, while joy calms it down to a regular wave.

Put simply, the MPA means standing back and observing your own thinking. As humans we can watch what we're saying, doing, thinking, feeling, and choosing, as well as our body language and even our intentions. When we do this, the front of the brain fires up, kindling a super healthy brain energy flow. More specifically, we get a great theta (healing and insight) and gamma (creativity, wisdom, learning, change) ratio.

> The MPA means standing back and observing your own thinking.

To control your thought life, you have to activate and continually make use of the quantum principle of *superposition*, which is the foundation of the MPA. Superposition is the ability to focus on incoming information: the external (what others are saying or doing; what you read, hear, or listen to; actions or events you witness; and so on) and the internal (upcoming thoughts from your nonconscious mind, your existing memories of all your life experiences, what you have learned, your nonconscious belief systems, your assumptions, and so on). In terms of cleaning up the mental mess, you need to train yourself to analyze this information in as objective a way as possible *before* you choose what to believe, what to reject, and what decisions to make.

What does superposition look like? Imagine sitting on a surfboard. A "magic" breeze is blowing through the networks of your mind as you're thinking, feeling, and choosing which way you want to tip the surfboard: either to ride the wave or to fall back and wait for the next one. It's as though time has frozen for a moment. This breeze makes you aware of some memories related to the current situation and your thinking patterns, preparing your brain to build a new memory. If you ask, answer, and discuss while in superposition, you're capturing your thoughts. It's almost as if you're watching yourself, becoming aware of what you're thinking and feeling, and focusing in as much detail as possible on the *now* moment—in the present.

For example, let's say you receive a text from someone challenging you about a belief you have, saying you're wrong. As you read the text (the incoming information), you'll be aware of a bunch of thoughts (internal information) related to this text message, such as your relationship to this person, your feelings of anger or irritation, and your beliefs. If you don't self-regulate your thinking, apply the 30–90 Second Rule, and get into the MPA, there's a strong chance you'll respond in frustration and use up valuable mental energy, which will make you even more upset. However, if you self-regulate your mind and use the 30–90 Second Rule and the MPA, you can stop yourself before you immediately text back. You can calm down enough to stand back or visualize yourself on that surfboard, acknowledging your feelings and deciding how you want to use your limited energy.

When you consciously engage with information that is coming into your brain in this way, you will be able to instinctively select around 15 to 35 percent of what you read, hear, and see, which is where the meaningful concepts are, while getting rid of the remaining 65 to 85 percent that is superfluous information. Essentially, when you use your MPA, your senses can tune in to the detail of the *now* moment—an enriching experience that will help you feel happier and more at peace. And, as you get into superposition using your MPA, you can choose to accept or override a thought. Remember, you have veto power over your thoughts when in superposition![4]

Mindfulness through practices such as meditation, yoga, and prayer allows you to develop a heightened sense of awareness in the present moment, accepting things as they are without judgment and emotional reactivity. Stepping into superposition using your MPA and the 5 Steps, you go *beyond mindfulness*. In this objective state, you're capturing and reconceptualizing toxic, chaotic thoughts and building healthy, organized thoughts. This is necessary to stabilize attention and develop habits you can actually use in your life.

So, the MPA helps you to intentionally shift your focus and observe your own mind-in-action in order to get multiple perspectives of the issue. It allows you to determine your own performance rather than get stuck replaying negative experiences in your head. The more you practice using your MPA, the more you won't be controlled by someone else's issues.

5. Boxes, Windows, Rewinding, and Suits of Armor

These visualization techniques are simple and fun directed neuroplasticity practices you can use in many ways both in the Neurocycle and as you go through the day. Visualizing is like daydreaming with a goal or a purpose.

a. *The Box Technique.* When people are really upsetting you, are toxic, or aren't respecting your boundaries, imagine putting them in a box. When they're in this box, you can't see or hear them, even though you might be looking at them or sitting next to them. This gives you the mental space to disconnect from their toxicity or emotional demands for a few moments while you catch your breath and decide how to respond.

b. *The Windows Technique.* Imagine a big building with lots of windows that are mostly sealed up. Put the toxic thought you're working on into one of the windows. Imagine you're on the outside of this window looking in. You can't climb into the window because it's inaccessible, but you have power over whatever is in that window. You are always safe where you're standing on the outside of the window—whatever is in that window cannot hurt you. You can embrace, process, and reconceptualize it whenever you're ready. Using the 5 Steps, you can visualize the

scene in the window changing as you reimagine it from a
safe distance.

c. *The Rewinding Technique.* This technique involves imagining that you're watching yourself in a movie. You have
control over each and every one of the scenes in this
movie. You can rewind and edit each scene using the 5
Steps. When you pause, you embrace your issue; when you
rewind, you process what is going on; when you replay,
you reconceptualize what you are thinking.

d. *The Suit of Armor Technique.* This visualization technique
is great for blocking toxic words coming at you from negative people. It helps to create a mental boundary to keep
your mental space safe. You do this by imagining you're
wearing a suit of armor. As the words hit you, they bounce
off you and back at the person. You don't have to process
and accept what they're saying. Instead, you deflect it.

Visualization helps to build the physical thought in the brain
prior to actually doing or saying whatever it is you need to do or say.
This means that when it comes to actually doing or saying something, you have already practiced it, so you're more prepared and
therefore more resilient and effective. In the case of using visualization in the above techniques, you're creating an imaginary scenario
that will help you calm down and regain control of your emotions.

All these directed neuroplasticity practices can be used in any
of the 5 Steps to help make embracing, processing, and reconceptualizing easier to manage.

6. Closing Your Eyes and Focusing on the Big Picture First

If something is very emotional, focusing first on the context, or
the big picture, takes a little of the sting out of it and also helps
with perspective and objectivity. This can make it easier to process
and find the root of the thought to reconceptualize it. For example,

let's say you are panicking about a loss of income. Rather than frantically getting stuck in the detail of all the financial implications, close your eyes and visualize what you could potentially do. Look at the impact of what you have already achieved and ask yourself questions like, *What is the overarching purpose of what I choose to do next? How can I do this in a scalable way to make an impact? How hard am I prepared to work to make this happen? What do I want to happen?*

Closing your eyes can help you gain perspective and channel your limited energy in an uplifting direction. Even closing your eyes for just a second can get you into the MPA mode of thinking, which will help calm you down, giving you the mental space to self-regulate your thinking and apply the 30–90 Second Rule.

Why? When you close your eyes, you tend to focus more on the big picture first, with less attention on the detail. Consciously focusing on the detail first when dealing with a toxic or challenging issue can be overwhelming, because it can lead to overgeneralizing and catastrophizing. In fact, it can cause cognitive inflexibility, rumination, and overthinking: you can't see the woods for the trees because you get so lost in all the details. We see this on the qEEG as red foci on the top of the head over an area called the *cingulate gyrus* (in the middle of the brain), which is active in an organized way when we're making use of our cognitive flexibility but is overactive when we are panicking.

Emotions activate bursts of high beta and gamma energy in the brain, as well as the release of serotonin, dopamine, and acetylcholine, which strengthen the load of the memory *if* you focus on the detail first. This is good if it's a healthy thought, but not so good if it's a toxic thought. Everything gets messy in a toxic situation. In the latter case, focusing on the big picture first can move this process in a positive direction, as I mentioned above, manipulating the energy in the brain, the neurochemicals, and the genetics of the brain to focus on the context of the thought. This, in turn, unblocks your thinking, kindling cognitive flexibility and bringing calm, insight, and perspective.[5] And the more you do this, the easier it gets.

The Discomfort Zones

There are physical, emotional, and informational warning signals from physical, emotional, and informational memories in a thought. Memories give off signals because they're dynamic and alive. They're very real and generate real energy. Emotional signals could be anything from anguish to joy; physical warning signals could be heart palpitations or GI symptoms, for example; an informational warning signal is the actual information that pops into your mind as a flashback.

There are four types of discomfort zones:

1. *The just aware zone*: prompts from the nonconscious to the subconscious mind, when you're just becoming aware of the physical sensations, feelings, and information of a thought. This is the *I can't quite put my finger on it, but something is worrying me* zone.

2. *The stress reaction zone*: physical warning signals from our body that something in our life needs to be addressed. When we make our stress work for us as a springboard into action, the sympathetic/parasympathetic nervous system and HPA axis are in balance. When we feel overwhelmed by our stress, these are out of balance and can make us feel physically ill. This is the *I feel a rush of adrenaline and my heart is really beating fast; something is really not right* zone.

3. *The emotional attitudes of the thought zone*: feelings of the thought that tell you something is off about a situation. This is the *I feel very wary and pushed in a corner; I am not comfortable* zone.

4. *The about-to-choose zone*: in superposition, holding multiple points of view in mind simultaneously as you consider the information in the thought. In this zone, you're thinking, *Okay, this situation needs to be analyzed carefully. I need to stop and take some time to think it through. This is my decision for now that I am comfortable choosing, and I won't proceed until I am comfortable and have peace.*

The simple flow diagram below gives you some examples of these emotional, physical, and informational warning signals. It's not exhaustive, but it will give you an idea of where to start and what to tune in to. The signals point to the *thought*, which, in turn, points to the thinking, feeling, and choosing that created the issue you're dealing with.

The warning signals, through the four discomfort zones, need to be embraced and processed, not suppressed. They're messengers, and you need to find the message. In the message is the solution. You need to accept the discomfort and mind-manage your way forward, by tiny steps, knowing that the brain is always changing no matter what you do, so you may as well control the change as much as you can.

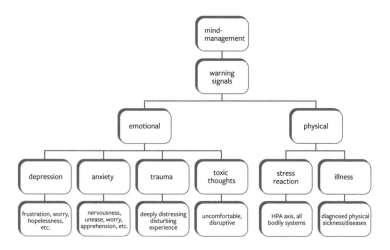

Emotional Warning Signals

Emotional warning signals are invitations to look inward. If you can't sit with them and listen to them, you run the risk of losing the opportunity to gain priceless information that will help with your healing.

Below is a simple, useful *emotional warning signal guide* to help you gauge where you're at, intensity-wise, as you use the 5-Step process. It's not a validated scale, just a simple guide to help you understand your level of intensity of whatever it is you're working on as you begin and then work through the 63-day cycle.

I want to, once again, stress that anxiety and depression are normal human reactions to things that are going on in our lives. They are words that are telling us to pay attention to something that's happening. They are not illnesses or diseases of the brain. Tuning in to your current emotions is part of the self-regulation process you are developing, which is essential to a mind-management lifestyle.

Preparing the Brain for Change

As I mentioned earlier, the 5 Steps should begin with a preparation phase, which involves calming and focusing exercises. This can

Some Emotions to Help Guide You

Today, I feel . . .

affection, anger, angst, anguish, annoyance, anxiety, apathy, arousal, awe, boredom, confidence, contempt, contentment, courage, curiosity, depression, desire, despair, disappointment, disgust, distrust, dread, ecstasy, embarrassment, envy, euphoria, excitement, fear, frustration, gratitude, grief, guilt, happiness, hatred, hope, horror, hostility, hurt, hysteria, indifference, interest, jealousy, joy, loathing, loneliness, love, lust, outrage, panic, passion, pity, pleasure, pride, rage, regret, relief, remorse, sadness, satisfaction, self-confidence, shame, shock, shyness, sorrow, suffering, surprise, terror, trust, wonder, worry, zeal, zest.

Emotional Warning Signal Guide

As you begin at day 1, step 1, you can do a quick level check on your emotions, note it in your diary, and track it as you begin to work through the 5 Steps each day. We all experience emotions and feelings in different ways under different circumstances—they can keep changing even in the space of one day or hour. Remember, there's nothing wrong with you if you feel you're at 7–10; you're simply experiencing something that needs attention.

Today, I feel . . .

1–3   Average. I have normal ups and downs as I go through life with all its challenges as a human in a complex world.

4–6   A hovering or floating anxiety and/or depression, worry, frustration, or toxic stress. I have that nagging angst that something is wrong but haven't quite pinpointed what yet. I understand it is more persistent because it often comes from stuff I have been suppressing just below the surface of my conscious awareness.

7–10 An increasing anxiety and/or depression that comes with not facing and dealing with stuff. I recognize this often explodes in different areas of life.

be breathing, meditation, tapping, mindful meditation, prayer, emotional freedom techniques, Havening, or any combination of these. I always begin with some preparation exercise, even if it's as simple as breathing in and out a few times to the count of three, because this aligns my mind-brain connection, facilitating the optimal flow of delta, theta, alpha, beta, and gamma in my brain, which, in turn, optimizes the physiology and DNA of the cells of my body and resets my brain at its deepest levels biochemically and electromagnetically.

Recent research has even shown that breathing, specifically exhaling, appears to be effective. As I mentioned earlier, my favorite is the Wim Hof method, because it's so scientific and works immediately.[6] The regular cycle of breathing is part of the mechanism that leads to conscious decision-making and acts of free will. So, when you do breathing exercises, not only do you calm down the parasympathetic and sympathetic nervous systems but you also gird up your decision-making capabilities. The point is to do whatever helps you get your mind focused in the moment and prepare your brain waves for the upcoming learning that will take place as you use the 5 Steps. This preparation stage increases the benefits of the Neurocycle exponentially. It also activates your neurotransmitters, resets the HPA axis, and primes the genes to respond in a more resilient way, which helps you develop a clearer and more resilient mind.

It's also important to note that a lot of unseen yet incredible brain, genetic, neuroendocrine, psychoneuroimmunological (mind-brain-immune system), and gut-brain things happen as we prepare the brain for deep thinking and deliberate learning. And, over time, these repeated exercises create habits, so if we practice enough we can get to a point where we can activate these breathing memories at will.

You can do any of these preparation strategies at any time for as long as you want, but in preparing to neurocycle, I would keep the preparation to anywhere between thirty seconds and three minutes. In my app, I have guided preparation exercises.

> *I have read several of your books, and have completed*
> *the 5 Steps, which has forever changed my life. Your*
> *work is refreshing, practical, applicable, and beneficial,*
> *refreshing the soul and mind. It makes me feel like*
> *I have some charge over my own destiny as I am*
> *responsible for what I am able. Thank you, Dr. Leaf.*
>
> VIVIAN

Chapter 10

Why It Takes Sixty-Three Days of Neurocycling to Form a Habit

<u>**Overview**</u>

- Building useful long-term thoughts into habits and detoxing toxic thoughts and traumas through directed neuroplasticity requires time and hard work and needs to be done regularly, as an ongoing process. When you finish working on one issue, you will begin working on the next issue—detoxing your mind is a lifestyle.

- Limit the time you spend detoxing toxic habits and trauma to around seven to thirty minutes a day because of the toll this process can have on you emotionally, mentally, and physically.

- You need to keep learning every day for mental health.

- We don't need to be held captive to our thoughts; instead, we can "capture" our thoughts!

- Whatever you experience in your mind will also be experienced in your brain and body. The toxic energy from toxic thoughts accumulates if it isn't dealt with, and will eventually explode in a volcanic and uncontrolled way.

> • Dealing with our toxic thoughts and traumas means that all this
>   swirling, chaotic, toxic energy needs to be transferred from the
>   negative thought to the reconceptualized, healthy thought to re-
>   store balance and coherence to the mind.

When I talk about neuroplasticity, I'm talking about how the mind changes the brain in energy, space, and time. We have already discussed how the mind changes the brain frequencies (*energy*) and also how it changes the brain's structure (*space*). The mind quite literally creates matter; that is, a new thought structure that changes the brain in a spatial way. There is one aspect we have not covered yet: how the mind changes the brain over *time*, and how this relates to the science of thought, the Neurocycle, brain-building, detoxing trauma, breaking down bad habits, and building good habits.

I'm not going to lie to you: building useful long-term thoughts into habits and detoxing toxic thoughts and traumas through directed neuroplasticity requires *time* and hard work and needs to be done regularly, as a lifestyle. We have to do something *more* than just read or listen to something once or twice or just work on an issue for a few days for real, sustainable, long-term change.

My research over the past three decades, including our recent clinical trial, shows that there's a time frame to mind-directed neuroplasticity, which we can use to guide and motivate us as we go *through* stuff and learn new information. As noted earlier, it takes around twenty-one days to build a long-term thought with its embedded memories, and sixty-three days to turn this thought into a habit. Along the way are specific time points (day 7, 14, 21, 42, and 63) where we feel changes happening, which can motivate us and help us get each thought that we're detoxing, or building, through this 63-day cycle. When it comes to the mind, it's the little, directed, and organized daily changes that cumulatively make the biggest difference.

So, when detoxing trauma (chapter 12) and breaking bad habits and building good ones (chapter 13), the 5 Steps should be done sequentially every day from day 1 to 21. From day 22 to 63, all you do is step 5, Active Reach. So, for the first twenty-one days you do active work, and for the forty-two days thereafter you practice the changes you've made. You can do this by adding your newly reconceptualized thought to the reminders on your phone, posting it on a sticky note, or whatever else works for you. You then simply read it to yourself to practice using the new way of thinking, which takes only a few seconds. The point is to remind yourself in a conscious and deliberate way every day. To be really effective in creating change, do the Active Reach at least seven times each day until day 63.

> It takes around twenty-one days to build a long-term thought with its embedded memories and sixty-three days to turn this into a habit.

For the first twenty-one days, I recommend taking around seven to thirty minutes total per day for all of the 5 Steps, or around one and a half to five minutes per step.

This is what it looks like:

Day 1

> Gather: 1.5–5 minutes
>
> Reflect: 1.5–5 minutes
>
> Write: 1.5–5 minutes
>
> Recheck: 1.5–5 minutes
>
> Active Reach: 1.5–5 minutes

Day 2–21: same timing as day 1

Day 22–63: about 1–7 minutes a day

Sometimes you may find you need a few cycles of sixty-three days—it will depend on what it is you are working on, how big the issue is, and what you're trying to change. Remember, each thought has a multitude of emotional, physical, and informational memories embedded in it, so thoughts are very complex, intertwined, and interconnected.

It will feel like you are working on multiple thoughts, but actually you are working on one thought that is problematic. Inside that thought are multiple memories, so you will have lots of memories in your mind as you are working on this thought. Remind yourself of the tree analogy: there are lots of branches representing what you are saying, doing, and feeling, which are coming from the root source. So, in essence, in the twenty-one days you will identify the thought with its memories and roots and reconceptualize it—not just replace it, which doesn't work. *Reconceptualizing* means finding the source/root/cause; identifying the mind-in-action that led to it; and changing this to include your story in a way you can handle (with the "sting" removed or neutralized), plus the new way you want to think about the situation that brings you peace. You then consciously practice using the new way of thinking for three to seven minutes a day (which is approximately the amount of time it takes to read the seven reminders of the Active Reach to bring it into your conscious awareness and apply it) for the next forty-two days—and you can start doing another 21-day cycle on a new toxic thought at the same time. Detoxing your mind is not a one-off event; it's a lifestyle.

Some helpful tips to keep you motivated through the sixty-three days:

1. Always remember there is a *defined and finite* time period: seven to thirty minutes per day at most.
2. Find an accountability partner.
3. Practice self-compassion and patience. Don't try to do too much in one day!

4. Make it fun. Tie in little rewards each day.
5. Remind yourself of the *physical* benefits from doing the mental work.
6. Look back at the review of my clinical trial to remind yourself of all the benefits of the 5 Steps.
7. This may be a good tool to use with your therapist if you have one.

It's important to limit the time you spend detoxing toxic habits and trauma to around seven to thirty minutes a day because of the toll this process can have on you emotionally, mentally, and physically. You don't want to be consumed by your issues, and if you spend too much time thinking about them you can get stuck in a sinking sand of toxic emotions and won't be able to function properly for the rest of the day. The 5 Steps are designed to give you structured, focused, and *time-restricted* mind/brain exercises to work on each day—and then you stop thinking about the toxicity of it for the rest of the day, except for your Active Reaches (step 5), which are positive pivots to a statement or simple action that will take only about a minute of your time to complete, and so are super easy but amazingly effective. This Active Reach step is designed to help you control your thinking and limit the emotional spillover into your day, which can occur when you are working on the hard stuff.

> When you are brain-building, you're not limited to seven to thirty minutes a day—you can spend as long as you want brain-building!

However, when you are brain-building (chapter 11), you're not limited to seven to thirty minutes a day—you can spend as long as you want brain-building! I typically try to spend at least two hours a day learning and building my brain (you will see how I do this in the daily mind-management plan in chapter 14). The brain-building process also works in

63-day cycles. However, for mental health, general resilience, and intelligence-building, this will look a little different. The 5 Steps of the Neurocycle should be done daily for at least thirty minutes, but you can go as long as you want. In these thirty or more minutes, you'll cycle through the 5 Steps with each chunk of information, which is about a paragraph of information. So, if the section of information you're learning (building as memories into your brain) is ten paragraphs, you'll do about ten neurocycles to build this into your brain. If you're studying for an exam, you'll neurocycle daily in preparation for the test. (I describe these latter processes in detail in my book *Think, Learn, Succeed*).

Throughout this brain-building process, it is important to remember that our mind and brain health depend on healthy, strong thoughts. When we stop learning and thinking deeply, we affect brain health, building up toxic waste in the brain. So, brain-building helps you with the harder work of detoxing. Just like not cleaning your teeth will affect your dental health, not learning can damage the brain, setting off a cascade of consequences. You need to keep learning every day for mental health.

> It's the little daily changes that cumulatively make the biggest difference.

As you build your brain and clean up your mental mess, it is also important to focus on other aspects of your lifestyle. I'll show you how eating, exercise, identity, connection, and sleep can also be addressed with the 5 Steps of mind-management. And as you do these daily over sixty-three days, you will be rewiring the brain in the direction you want it to go.

Benchmark Days in the 63-Day Cycle

As you go through this 63-day process, there are benchmark days that can motivate you and help you get through the thought you're detoxing or building. These specific benchmarks are at days 7, 14,

21, and 63. Knowing a little about the timing of these benchmarks and what's happening in your brain at each one can help you push through the hard times and achieve true and lasting change in your life as you use the 5 Steps, just as seeing the difference in your body after a hard training regimen can motivate you to continue on.

On **day 1,** you'll experience a type of apprehensive excitement as conscious awareness builds with self-regulation and awareness. At first, the prefrontal cortex (executive function) has controlled high-beta bursts of energy as you begin to focus and a nice pattern of low-beta as your awareness increases. The amygdala (emotional perceptions) and hippocampus (memory conversion) have a lot of low-beta energy and coherent bursts of high-beta, theta, and gamma as thoughts with embedded memories are being recalled—even delta is high as suppressed thoughts are being activated. Then, as processing takes place, gamma increases and peaks, which means learning begins taking place a little each day (the neuroplastic changes happening in the brain). You're starting to positively affect the architecture of the brain—you're starting to push the structural changes in your brain in the direction you want them to go.

By **day 4,** the increased awareness from the work you're doing on your thoughts, which is very challenging to say the least, increases your sense of autonomy, which can also increase your stress levels because you're starting to face some potentially hard issues. This is understandable because you're literally drawing up established thoughts with their embedded informational and emotional memories from the nonconscious, and this is hard work—even a little scary. But rest assured, your nonconscious mind has the wisdom to know how much you can handle. This is also the reason that you spend only thirty minutes maximum per day on detoxing. Day 4 sees increases in alpha, theta, and delta in the brain in response to you feeling a little anxious and even fearful, as it's tough facing stuff, but I remind you again that you have enough wisdom to know how much you can handle.

By **day** 7, you'll have a sense of insight and satisfaction and a sense of *This is going somewhere.* You'll be starting to realize that there's hope and that you do have a sense of control. You'll begin to feel empowered and even excited. This increases your alpha and gamma. Deep inside your brain, there are amazing structural changes happening—you'll be growing little bumps on your dendrites, like those little bumps of leaf buds on branches of a tree. This means your memories are being processed and reconceptualized—change is happening! Look at the dendrite image below; on the branch that has three shapes on it, look at the circular bump—that's what is happening on hundreds, maybe even thousands, of your dendrites.

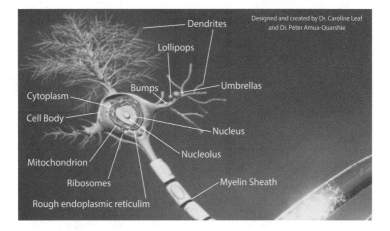

Designed and created by Dr. Caroline Leaf and Dr. Peter Amua-Quarshie

By **day 14,** you'll have a definite sense of achievement; you will feel like *I've got this!* But be careful. Often this is when people stop, as they think that they've done all the work because it feels like things are under control. But you can't stop here! It's important to use this sense of achievement to propel yourself forward, not to rest on your laurels. Remember, complacency stunts growth and progress. The bumps on the dendrites have changed to lollipop shapes, demonstrating the neuroplasticity of the brain, and the delta, theta, alpha, beta, and gamma are flowing in a nice, regulated pattern, which contributes to this sense of achievement. Look at the dendrite image again to see the lollipop next to the bump.

By **day 21,** you will feel a strong sense of resolve, commitment, and determination that *This is hard, but I can do this. I now understand that the toxic emotions are not scary but actually my route to freedom. It's okay if I have bad days, because this is a normal human reaction to the challenges of life. I know what to do with these signals now.* You and others will see and experience the changes in you, which is really motivating. In the brain, there will be a mix of all frequencies, with bursts of high beta, which reflect a little bit of controlled anxiety. There will also be gamma peaks, which show the neuroplastic changes that have resulted in the newly reconceptualized thought. On the dendrites, the lollipops change into mushroom shapes as the proteins become self-sustainable, which means they're strong enough to hold the energy of memories of the thought for the long-term. Look back at the image to see the mushroom shape next to the lollipop.

Days 22 to 63 will bring a sense of peace and a mature realization that depression and anxiety are signals to be used to your advantage to find and change your reactions. Theta and delta will increase in activity as habit formation occurs. By day 63, when automatization happens (the thought moves into the nonconscious as a habit and works to influence your behavior) you will have a sense of empowerment and overall well-being as you realize you can't control the events and circumstances that led to the feelings of depression, or whatever else you were experiencing, but you *can* learn to embrace them in order to change and control your reactions.

Over each 63-day cycle, the 5 Steps will increase your sense of autonomy and feeling of control. This, in turn, will lead to increased awareness of and the ability to deal with your toxic thoughts, which will help you control toxic stress and change your perspective about how you're looking at the world. You'll start seeing challenges and barriers as opportunities, feel more in control, and have more overall life satisfaction. The 5 Steps of mind-management literally provide a pathway to empowerment.

If you really want to have mental peace, dealing with past traumas or toxic thought habits is necessary. You have to strategically, proactively, deliberately, and intentionally self-regulate how you think, feel, and choose, building healthy thoughts while detoxing unhealthy ones. Considering that unhealthy thoughts cause brain damage, doesn't this seem like a worthwhile pursuit?

The Science behind Using the Neurocycle over Sixty-Three Days

The moment you wake up in the morning, the conscious mind comes online, as seen by increased beta activity in brain scans. And, as you move into the process of "awake neuroplasticity"— thinking, feeling, and choosing to build thoughts—you're changing the structure of your brain very rapidly. Considering you are always thinking (even when you are sleeping, your mind is sorting out the thoughts it has built during the day), and the brain is *always* changing because it's neuroplastic, you may as well proactively and strategically take control of this process and drive neuroplasticity in the direction you want it to go.

As you experience life, the structure of the DNA changes in response, like playdough. This means genes that were hidden before become exposed, which is how gene activity is regulated and proteins are made and form into dendritic branches, and a thought tree grows in the brain.[1] If it's a healthy experience, there will be healthy gene activity; if the experience is negative, there will be a gene mutation and the dendritic branches will be toxic. This is the plastic paradox: the brain and body can change, but in both a negative or a positive direction. The good news is that you can always change negatives back to positives.

Remember, neuroplastic change, whether in a negative or a positive direction, also follows a definitive time line. I can't say this often enough: it takes twenty-one days to build a long-term thought and then another forty-two days to automatize that thought. An automatized thought is one that impacts your behavior, and therefore we can say it's a habit. That is why it takes sixty-three days to form a habit.

> Neuroplastic change, whether in a negative or positive direction, also follows a definitive time line.

As you think, feel, and choose in response to the experiences of life (which you are doing all day long—you never stop, not even for three seconds), quantum waves of energy activity flood the brain. Your mind-in-action dictates the shape, intensity, and impact of these waves (we can pick this up on a qEEG), which in turn influence the biochemistry of the brain and body.

These waves of energy stimulate computational activity in the cell bodies of neurons (see image below), like a computer. The connection (synaptic) strength between neurons increases the more focused and deep your thinking, feeling, and choosing are, because this causes repeated firing of synapses; that is, high-frequency stimulation and lots of buzz at the synapses. This is called long-term potentiation (LTP), which is short-term memory that has the *potential* to become long-term memory if you focus repeatedly on the information for at least twenty-one days. If not, then the short-term memory only lasts for about twenty-four to forty-eight hours. For example, say you read a great article on something interesting; three days or a week later, you'll remember you read the article and the big picture of what it was about, but you'll find you have forgotten most of the details

However, if you do something with this thought, such as deeper and more deliberate thinking, you will activate and upregulate

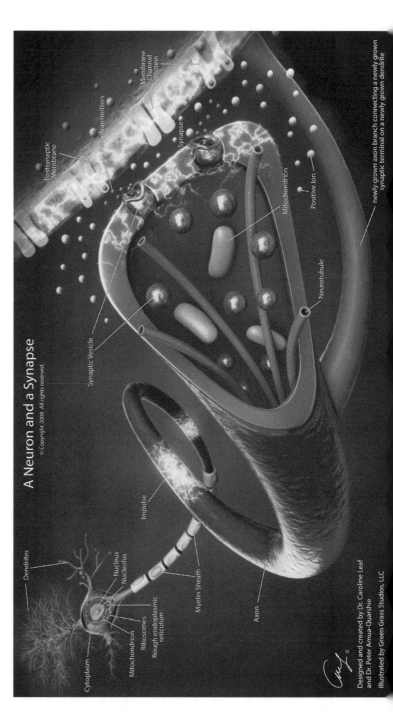

A Neuron and a Synapse

Dendrites

Nucleus
Nucleolus

Cytoplasm

Mitochondrion
Ribosomes
Rough endoplasmic
reticulum

Myelin Sheath

Impulse

Axon

Designed and created by Dr. Caroline Leaf
and Dr. Peter Amua-Quarshie
Illustrated by Green Grass Studios, LLC

Postsynaptic
Membrane

Neurotransmitters

Synapse

Membrane
Channel
Protein

Mitochondrion

Positive Ion

Neurotubule

Synaptic Vesicle

newly grown axon branch connecting a newly grown
synaptic terminal on a newly grown dendrite

gene activity and cause the dendrites (the tops of the neurons—see the image above) to grow, which is where thoughts eventually configure into long-term thoughts with embedded memories as quantum vibrations in tiny protein "quantum computers," called *tubulin*, form from the increased gene activity. It takes at least twenty-one days of daily work to build up enough energy to create long-term memory. The more you practice deliberate, self-regulatory thinking by using a mind-management process like the 5 Steps, the more energy you are giving the thought—like watering a plant. Remember, whatever you think about the most will grow.

If you daily, regularly think in this deliberate, deep, and focused way over the twenty-one days, you are feeding the dendrites energy, and they will start to grow bumps, called spines, around day 7, which means the thought is getting stronger.[2] These look a bit like the nodes on a branch when a new branch forms on a tree (see the dendrite image). This kind of focused mind action involves becoming aware of how you are feeling mentally and physically, standing back and observing your own thinking, capturing these thoughts, and processing and reconceptualizing them.

These bumps on the dendrites change shape over time in response to *daily*, *deep*, *deliberate* thinking. The bump means the memory is still quite weak and vulnerable. But as you think and focus daily on the thought in a regular and deliberate way, the bump becomes a lollipop shape on the dendrite around day 14, which means the thought is getting stronger.

- As you continue to do daily mind work on the thought, the lollipop shape changes to a mushroom shape on the dendrite around day 21, becoming more self-sustainable with stronger proteins and energy, which give the thought longevity. So, a long-term thought with its embedded memories (emotional, informational, physical) looks like more and more mushroom-shaped spines on the dendrites. Long-term thoughts, *not habits*, are formed around the

21-day mark. The energy generated by this process includes beta and theta waves, with gamma peaks flowing from the front to the back of the brain at forty times per second.[3] We saw this happening with the subjects in our research study between days 7 and 21, as the subjects were embracing, processing, and reconceptualizing their toxic stress.

- From days 22 to 63, more mind work needs to be done to turn the long-term thought into a habit.[4] Habits are basically thoughts that are accessible and usable and that manifest as changes in what you say and do. A simple example is learning to drive a car—as you learn, you're building the thoughts. Eventually, you know how to drive after learning the basics, then you practice using this knowledge. One day you just get in the car and drive, seemingly without thinking. How? You're driving from the useful thought trees of driving you have built into your brain as a habit (a useful and accessible memory). The dendrites built over the twenty-one days need more energy to grow their strength in order to be able to make an impact on your behavior—they need to be fed energy (practice) to grow into accessible and useful thoughts (habits). Extra gamma peaks occur at day 21 and again at day 42, which are needed for habits to form—without these extra peaks, habits won't form and the long-term thought with its embedded memories won't be accessible. The knowledge you need won't be at your fingertips, and the changes you are trying to make won't be seen or experienced. The energy needed to make a memory accessible and useful is coming from your mind through practicing the new way of thinking—exactly like you practice a new skill like driving. Again, for twenty-one days you *build* a new thought, then for another forty-two days you *practice* using what you have built. This type of useful and accessible thought gives you that edge that enables you to, for example, talk intelligently about that article you just read or podcast you just listened to, recall those facts during that business meeting, debate, or exam, or—drive that car!

So, what is *forgetting*? Forgetting can happen anywhere along the 63-day cycle. If you don't think as deeply or regularly about something, or if you stop thinking about it completely, the synapse will lose energy and strength. As a result, the proteins around the sensitive synapse will disappear, causing a decrease in dendritic spines and dendrites; the tiny proteins holding the memories will denature (die off), and you will forget about the thing or experience. Your thoughts literally convert to hot air!

And this means change won't happen in your life, and you will feel frustrated because you keep starting to change but don't carry it through to the end—sixty-three days at least. It's incredibly important to remember that whether information gets stored in the dendrites or not depends on *how intentionally you think about something*; that is, how much time and effort you expend thinking about it.

And this is what the 5 Steps train you to do. You can think of the mind-management that happens though neurocycling like this: as you think you are *feeding* the memory, and this food is either junk food, which makes a mess, or healthy food, which is nourishing and leads to clarity. What we remember, learn, and change is in our hands. That's a very powerful and sobering thought.

This also means that if you stop feeding the thought with its embedded memories, you'll forget most of it. That's great if it's a bad thought but bad if it's a good thought. You have to keep at it until it gets automatized, which is when the energy will stabilize and become useful to you. If you stop working on something at any point in the 63-day cycle, you've stopped feeding the thought. No food means no energy, which means the thought disappears and you're back to square one, repeating the same bad habits and getting stuck in the same toxic patterns. By the same token, you can feed a *toxic thought* and make it grow even more toxic over the sixty-three days—and consequently build a toxic habit. As mentioned earlier, this is called the *plastic paradox*, because now you've used your neuroplasticity to make your thoughts even more toxic.

You need to push yourself to get to the highest level of thought, which involves facing *and* pushing through adversity, and therefore channeling your energy. This type of thinking builds strong dendrites with mushroom spines, which are long-term memories that are coherent, with balanced theta and gamma working in synchrony.

○ ○ ○ ○

In summary, in order for a memory to be *usable*, it needs lots of energy. It gets lots of packets of energy (*quanta*) when you repeatedly think about the memory daily, through the disciplined process of going through all 5 Steps of mind-management very systematically for the first twenty-one days, which facilitates the required neurochemical and structural changes in the brain that make this memory a usable and useful thought. Then, for the next forty-two days, you consciously practice using the new thought, which allows a useful *habit* to form. When a thought becomes accessible, it informs your next decision, such as knowing the answer on an exam or what to say to that person who upset you. If you do not automatize the memory, however, it will not be accessible and, therefore, not be helpful to you.

Unfortunately, most people give up within the first week of learning or trying to change a toxic habit or fix a trauma. As a result, they have to start all over again, which isn't only tedious and disheartening but also creates negative feedback loops in the brain and body. Quick fixes and memory tricks are illusions—don't let them fool you. Trust the science!

○ ○ ○ ○

Remember, the Neurocycle is a way to harness your thinking power; any task that requires thinking can use it, which means everything can— because you're always thinking! In the next few chapters, we're going to discuss how to use the 5 Steps to manage our minds, no matter what we're doing or changing. But, before we dive in, I want to briefly explain how the rest of of the book is laid out.

First, you'll learn how to use the 5 Steps to build your brain and develop mental toughness and brain health. This is an ongoing, daily task to clean up your mental mess, much like the daily routine we have to keep ourselves and our living spaces clean. Next, you'll learn how to neurocycle to detox trauma from your mind and brain. This is like a deep clean, like when you have to move things out of the way in your home to clean behind the furniture and scrub the mold out from between the shower tiles.

Then we'll learn how to break bad habits and build good lifestyle habits. This is like a spring clean, where you get rid of the old and bring in the new and freshen up the look of your home—or, in this case, your mind. I've also included a few neurocycle life hacks to help you handle basic, everyday scenarios like dealing with toxic people or people-pleasing.

Part 2 ends with a daily mind-management plan, which is my fail-safe routine to keep my mind regulated and my brain clean— this will pull everything together, helping you adapt the 5-Step process to your unique lifestyle.

Dr. Leaf! It is so very, very exciting for me to discover that I am finding my "thinker" again. By using your mental management techniques, I have been working at what I call "building bridges" over the black holes of my mind (the places where I would literally go blank in my thinking. I have multiple white matter deficits in my brain MRI . . . and I call these areas my "black holes" because I can literally feel when I drop into cognitive confusion in one of these areas). I had been learning to live with these deficits, and to try to get on with life with cognitive disabilities. But now, I truly believe that I have learned tools to help rebuild my brain and rebuild my memory, and perhaps one day, I will once again feel confident in my cognitive skills.

KELLY

Chapter 11

Neurocycling to Build Your Brain and Develop Mental Toughness

The mind is just like a muscle—the more you exercise it, the stronger it gets and the more it can expand.

Idowu Koyenikan

The brain is in love with the mind. As you think, you're using your mind to change the microscopic structure of your brain. With every experience, your mind is causing real-time chemical and structural changes in the brain. Mind changes matter literally instantaneously. As you read in the section on neuroplasticity, the brain isn't a fixed lump of matter delivering genetically preprogrammed instructions to the body. Rather it's an intensely responsive and intricately complex, constantly changing system of cells, and *we*, using our mind, are the cause of the changes. The brain is hungry for and *needs* these changes. In fact, the brain can't *not* change—and as we all know, when our minds are a mess for whatever reason life throws at us, the changes in the brain can go awry pretty quickly. However, there's something we can do to help the brain function well and build resilience against the challenges of life: brain-building. We need to use our mind to build or "feed" our brain regularly, just like we need to eat regularly. Brain-building is like eating a healthy diet. It's a process of "feeding" the brain regularly with new and challenging information (healthy food) that is well "digested," meaning it's deeply understood.

The process of brain-building is rapid. Genes are activated within a few minutes, and a single neuron may gain thousands of new dendritic branches in a very short time.

In fact, brain-building is so important that it's one of the first things I would train my patients to do, whatever their specific need was. It's a powerful tool; my early research showed up to 75 percent improvement in academic, cognitive, social, emotional, and intellectual function when people were taught how to build their brain and harness deep, intellectual thought. When you build your brain, you build your resilience and your intelligence. This changes the way that energy flows through the brain, optimizing its function and cognitive flexibility. Brain-building also uses the thousands of new baby nerve cells that are born when we wake up each morning, called *neurogenesis*. If we don't use these baby nerve cells and don't brain-build, toxic waste builds up in the brain that will affect our mood and sleep and will lower the resilience of the brain, increasing our vulnerability to mental and physical issues.

I brain-build every day without fail, along with detoxing my thoughts. I even use brain-building to help calm and refocus my mind in the midst of a panic or anxiety attack or if I'm worried about something. Brain-building is, I believe, one of the most powerful resilience-building mental health tools out there, and completely underrated in the wellness industry.

Don't get me wrong; "fixing" toxic thoughts with their embedded emotions is huge, and I'll help you deal with this in the next chapter. However, what we often don't speak about is how we need strong, optimized brains and clear, intelligently functioning minds to *do* the work of "fixing." Through brain-building you can achieve this, which is why it's a huge part of the mind-management process.

> Brain-building is one of the most powerful resilience-building mental health tools out there.

Perhaps brain-building doesn't get enough attention because it's not as "glamorous" as a pill or new, trendy workout. Additionally, brain-building takes a long time, and the results aren't immediately seen. Yet without a strong brain we cannot have sustainable improvements in our physical and mental health, just like an old, damaged car cannot go any faster or be any better even if you put in the best quality fuel.

Brain-building is, quite simply, using the 5 Steps in an organized way to learn new information—directed neuroplasticity at its finest! This can be any information that grabs your interest or that you need to master for school or work. The information needs to be learned with the goal of understanding it deeply enough to be able to teach it to a class, have an intelligent discussion on the topic, or write an exam on the information (preferably all of these). Not only will this exercise increase your brainpower and intelligence but it will also activate resilience in your mind and brain, which will equip you to manage your emotions and think more effectively and with more clarity.

And, as a bonus during tough times, it buys you time to calm down when you're worked up. As mentioned above, I would do this with my patients first thing. We would literally start with brain-building their schoolwork or studying an article they were interested in—and only when they felt strong enough did we tackle their "heavy stuff." It's not distracting you from dealing with the hard stuff; it's preparing you to be uncomfortable enough to change.

There's another great benefit to brain-building: it's a neuro-plasticity-driven system that keeps the brain tidy and clean. It helps transfer chaotic and messy mental energy to organized mental energy, like when we vacuum up dirt and clean our homes to get some level of order back.

> Brain-building is a neuroplasticity-driven system that keeps the brain tidy and clean.

When you brain-build, you introduce a level of control, which helps you feel hope again. This may be only a glimmer of hope at first, but it's there! The boxes are now neatly packed in your closet; they're filled with stuff that still needs organizing, but at least they aren't all over the floor! You have prioritized them and created some sort of order.

Brain-building is also a great way to help reduce sleeping issues. If you find yourself struggling to fall asleep or waking up because of anxious thoughts, you may have too much "toxic buildup" in your brain from unused neurons. By building your brain, you use these neurons in a healthy way throughout the day so at night they don't emerge with a vengeance, begging to be used and heard.

Here is one more reason why brain-building is amazing and so vital: it can help you get "unstuck" in any area of life, such as in a job, in a relationship, or with a project. When feeling stuck, try the following brain-building boosters:

1. Question how high your bar for originality is. Keep in mind there is nothing new, just new ways of saying things. As you read and learn more, you'll realize there are common messages throughout; people just say them in different and unique ways.

2. Have an *experimental* mindset, which means to explore, test, analyze results, pivot if it doesn't work, and repeat.

3. Be an infinite learner always. Read fiction *and* nonfiction (fiction is especially great for boosting creativity and problem-solving abilities), listen to podcasts, engage in tough conversations, travel.

4. Be open to any and all opportunities. *Be open to the yes.* If something sounds remotely interesting, pursue it.

5. Don't fall into the trap of having to be great at something to try it. Embrace the opportunity to learn. Remember: every great athlete was not great in the beginning and had to learn.

6. Be prepared to have those difficult conversations—you can learn so much from these. Get comfortable agreeing to disagree.

Using the Neurocycle for Brain-Building

Here's a simple overview for how to use the 5 Steps of the Neurocycle for brain-building. If you really want to get into the nitty gritty of how to use brain-building on a whole other level to improve grades and thrive in the workplace and life, I recommend my book *Think, Learn, Succeed.*

1. **Gather.** The goal of the Gather step is straightforward: to understand what you're hearing, reading, and experiencing, and to get the information into the brain properly. As you go through this step, it's important to remember we are thinking beings; we think all day long.

   Choose the information you're going to practice brain-building with. This could be this book, an article in a magazine, something in your newsfeed, a YouTube video, an audiobook, or a podcast—anything that contains information that challenges and interests you. Now, read a paragraph or a small section of two or three sentences, or listen to a minute or so of the audio. Then stop and go to step 2.

2. **Reflect.** The aim of this focused thinking step is to learn how to think deeply and intentionally, which will develop your phenomenal capacity to build effective, long-term memory into your dendrites. The Golden Rule of the 5 Steps is to *think to understand* the information you're trying to remember, which involves three steps: asking, answering, and discussing.

   - *Ask* yourself what you've read—the who, what, when, where, why, and how.

   - *Answer* by reviewing what you've just read or heard, re-reading the chunk of information out loud and circling around 15–35 percent of the concepts, or rewatching/relistening to the video/audio and writing down around 15–35 percent of what you see or hear. Don't underline or highlight words—these are passive actions and don't require you to think, analyze, or understand. Circling and thinking about each chunk is more active.

   - *Discuss* this chunk of information with yourself while still looking at the material. Explain it to yourself over and over in your own words until you understand it. If you can't work out what it means, ask someone or make a note to find out later. Really interact with the material. To get into the habit of doing so, ask yourself about the information, answer yourself by paraphrasing what you've read or heard, and discuss it with yourself. This interaction allows the nerve cells to switch on the gene that makes strong, long-term memories grow in the dendritic branches.

3. **Write.** This step involves writing down the information you selected in the analytical thinking step above. I recommend you use the "brain-friendly" way of writing I have

created, called the Metacog (see appendix B). It's really important to write concepts down as you do the ask/answer/discuss process, because this reinforces healthy dendrite growth and really forces you to think about your thinking. Remember, the brain operates like a quantum computer. As you think (step 2), you create signals in your brain; as you write words down in a brain-friendly format, you reinforce and strengthen these quantum signals and what you have just grown in the dendrites. You're literally influencing your genetic expression and growing your brain.

4. **Recheck** helps build useful long-term memory into the dendrites. It's a very simple yet extremely powerful process. All you have to do is deliberately and intentionally go through what you've written, either in your journal or on your Metacog, to see if it makes sense, and if it has all the necessary information on it. It goes without saying that you can't learn from something that doesn't make sense to you, and the Recheck step helps with this. It involves a cross-evaluation of the content of your written work.

   How to do the Recheck step:

   1. Make sure you understand what you've written. Sort the information out to understand it, then compare it to the original content for accuracy.

   2. Make certain you're satisfied with the information you have selected, which will be in concept form.

   3. Look for whether you have too much or too little information using the 15–35 percent guideline.

   4. Ask yourself if the Metacog makes sense, and if it doesn't, edit it until it does.

   5. Check whether you have organized the information in a logical way.

   6. Check for cross-linking of information.

7. Check if you can make the concepts easier to remember by adding more pictures, symbols, or color, or maybe even deleting some words or images.

8. Repeat steps 1–4 until you've finished the information you're learning. You might do this process over a few days before you actually get to step 5, which happens once you have completed a section—the video, podcast, chapter of the book you're reading, and so on.

5. **Active Reach.** In this step, you play "teacher" and sequentially reteach all the information that's on your Metacog. Teach it to your dog, your cat, or whoever will listen to you! You can even reteach yourself in the mirror. Explain what you're learning out loud. Using all of your senses will make your brain work harder and build the memory more effectively. Test yourself in some way; perhaps create some questions you think may be asked by your boss or teacher. Ask yourself questions that will help you apply the information to your life in a real and tangible way.

The mental practice that happens in this active stage strengthens existing new dendrites and increases the spines on the outside of the dendrites.

How to do the Active Reach:

- Reteach the information in a way that you would like to have had it explained to you, or as though you're explaining it in a second language. This involves explaining what you've learned carefully, in multiple ways and in detail, elaborating by way of extra examples.

- Imagine and see this as though watching a movie of what you are learning. Paint a picture in your mind of the information, which makes it come alive. Research has shown that imagination leads to physical changes in the memory.

- Look for trigger words, phrases, or images that bring back whole chunks of information to your mind.
- Ask yourself what the author is trying to tell you in order to understand the meaning behind what you're reading.

I want to say thank you for helping to change my life, my mind, my brain, and now my ability to help other therapists in our coaching practice!

AMY

Chapter 12

Neurocycling to Detox Trauma

A vast majority of the collective is traumatized. It's our secret, unrecognized epidemic. Trauma extends far beyond the "big" events. At its core it's disconnection from true self. It presents as depression, deep loneliness, and anxiety. All of us have healing to do. All of us are guiding each other home—back to the mind, body, spiritual connection we had at birth. "Broken" is the illusion created by trauma. Wholeness is the truth.

DR. NICOLE LePERA

Overview

- When you find yourself becoming defensive or trying to distract away the awareness, *lean in to what you may be trying to avoid*. It will be ugly and messy, but if you don't address it, it will just stay ugly and messy.
- Toxic trauma involves something that happened to us that was out of our control, and often results in a pervasive feeling of threat. It includes things like adverse childhood experiences, traumatic experiences at any age, war trauma, and all forms of abuse, including racial aggression and socioeconomic oppression.

- Trauma is probably the hardest thought pattern to work on, which is why so many therapists and counselors spend years working on trauma with their clients. Toxic trauma requires a lot of work, time, grace, and self-compassion, as it involves embracing, processing, and reconceptualizing things that are generally incredibly painful and upsetting.
- An acute situation is an unforeseen and unwelcome event that can blindside us, is often traumatic, and can throw our brains and bodies into crisis mode.
- The Neurocycle is not designed to remove all our suffering. Rather, it helps us reconceptualize it, which is to view a memory from a new perspective so we no longer feel pain when we think about something that previously caused us emotional distress.
- You can *pretrain* your mind to embrace and deal with the panic and anxiety acute situations bring.
- Doing something reactively under such conditions very often makes things worse, leading to more anxiety and the breakdown of any actions that are in fact appropriate to dealing with the actual threat.
- We have the power to control our reactions in this moment as we draw on the wisdom of the nonconscious mind to manage a crisis.

This chapter will cover how to neurocycle to detox trauma. Trauma comes in three forms: acute trauma, big "T" trauma, and little "t" trauma.

Acute Trauma

An acute trauma is sudden such as unexpected illnesses, pandemics, wars, death, a financial crisis, job loss, car accidents, extreme weather conditions, racially charged attacks, or unexpected problems with family members. Acute situations put our body on high alert in order to cope with a sudden change. This can be good for us, as it prepares the body to act in the face of danger. However, if we mismanage the situation, we can shift into toxic stress, which can have negative physical and mental repercussions. For example, when we're in a toxic stress state, our blood vessels around the heart constrict and there will be less blood flow and oxygen to the brain, putting the brain and heart at risk for a stroke or cardiac event.

I personally experienced acute trauma when my son, Jeffrey, was brutally attacked while on a study abroad program in Rome. He was on the phone with me as it happened—I was in Washington, DC, for a conference—and the phone just went dead. For two hours after the incident we didn't know if he was even alive.

In the moment, the shock made me feel like I was dying. I had to make some quick life-or-death decisions to protect him, and I needed my mind to be strong enough to do so in that moment. After doing the 5 Steps of mind-management, I was able to stop, breathe, and call my husband and several friends I knew in Italy and Europe, one of whom I knew had a contact in the Italian police.

Acute trauma is usually brief, though its repercussions can last a long time. It throws our brains and bodies into crisis mode, which, if mind-managed with the Neurocycle, can work for us even if it is still incredibly painful and traumatic. Unmanaged acute trauma can accelerate post-traumatic stress and lead to increased risk for depression and anxiety—and to poor decision-making at the worst possible time.

That's why we need to be *proactive* in training our mind and brain to be ready, because we never know when a crisis may hit. Though we can't control the events and circumstances that lead to an acute situation, we can take control of our reactions in order to best manage them. In this instance the 5 Steps are like insurance.

> Acute trauma is usually brief and throws our bodies and brains into crisis mode.

I guarantee that when a crisis comes along, you'll be glad to have a bulletproof plan to not only help with the stressful event but also manage afterward and prevent toxic coping habits from forming. You are pretraining your brain and increasing your resilience.

When my son was being attacked in Rome, I cried and felt terrified and fearful. But I also immediately started working toward what I could do.

1. **I did my *preparation*.** I used the box method for breathing to calm my mind: I breathed in for four counts, held for four counts, breathed out for four counts, held for four counts. I repeated this three or four times.

   You could also try this helpful grounding technique exercise, which will help center your mind when things feel overwhelming and stressful:

   1. Acknowledge five things you see around you.
   2. Acknowledge four things you can you touch around you.
   3. Acknowledge three things you can hear.
   4. Acknowledge two things you can smell.
   5. Acknowledge one thing you can taste.

2. **I started using the 5 *Steps of the Neurocycle***

   1. *Gather.* I gathered awareness of my racing thoughts and physical stress reactions.
   2. *Reflect.* I reflected on how I was losing control and starting to say negative things, and how this was blocking my ability to decide what to do. I reflected on the fact that I was frozen on the floor sobbing in panic. I closed my eyes and started focusing on the big picture and context, and told myself and my daughter, who was with me, that his friends would bring help, the teachers would find him, or someone would

help him. I prayed for his protection, drawing on my knowledge of quantum physics and spirituality.

3. *Write.* I mentally grabbed those negative thoughts that were freezing me. I refused to let my brain's neuroplasticity go in that direction and forced myself to say three positive statements for every negative statement that came into my mind—out loud.

4. *Recheck.* I reconceptualized the toxic thought *Is he dead?* that was crippling me into a memory verse I had learned as a child: *He will live and not die.* I repeated this over and over while breathing in and out rhythmically to the count of three to calm my HPA axis down.

5. *Active Reach.* I channeled my panic into action and called my husband, Mac, who immediately called a security friend with global connections, and a whole cycle of events was put into motion to find and save my son. In the meantime, we called family and close friends, and each person was soon doing something with us to try to solve the problem—from tracing Jeffrey's cell phone to praying to calling contacts in Rome to speaking to the police to contacting the head of the study abroad program in Rome.

I had to neurocycle over and over with different objectives as we waited in agony for news. It kept me focused and able to be effective in the midst of my panic.

Finally, two hours later, Jeffrey called. In a broken voice, he told us he had managed to crawl to a café, and the people working there had called the police, and he had then gone for an emergency checkup at the hospital before being taken back to his school.

Then the long road to healing began as we dealt with the immediate acute trauma and the post-trauma, which was a big

"T": the nightmares, the fears, and the anxiety. Jeffrey, my other three children, my husband, and I had to embrace, process, and reconceptualize this trauma over the next few months together. Facing the pain and pushing through it with people we love and trust is the only way to get through—we aren't meant to do it alone!

The feeling of being out of control is the pulse of acute trauma and is, without doubt, extremely disconcerting. We naturally want to protect ourselves and our loved ones. It all feels *too much*, which is why we need mind-management to stop from drowning. When everything around us feels completely chaotic and unmanageable, the 5 Steps can be our life vest.

Big "T" Trauma and Little "t" Trauma

Toxic trauma involves something that happened to us that was out of our control and often results in a pervasive feeling of threat. It includes things like adverse childhood experiences, traumatic experiences at any age, war trauma, and all forms of abuse, including racial aggression and socioeconomic oppression. The experience of trauma is vastly different for each person, and the healing process is also different. There's no magic solution that can help everyone, and it takes time, work, and the willingness to face the uncomfortable for true healing to take place, as hard as this can be. Thankfully, there's no deadline when it comes to overcoming trauma—you do it in a way that works for you.

Trauma has a different pattern in the mind and brain than a toxic habit, which we will learn about in the next section, does. It's involuntary and has been inflicted on a person, which often leaves the person feeling emotionally and physically exposed, worn out, and fearful. Trauma is probably the hardest thought pattern to work on, which is why so many therapists and counselors spend years working on trauma with their clients. Toxic trauma requires a lot of work, time, grace, and self-compassion, as it involves embracing, processing, and reconceptualizing things that are generally incredibly painful and upsetting.

Everyone has some level of trauma to work on, whether it's big "T" trauma of something profoundly disturbing, like war or rape, or something more commonplace but still very serious, like bullying or trying to help a loved one suffering through an illness. All trauma needs attention, regardless of what its root is, because trauma by its very nature is pervasive and destructive to our sense of mental peace and happiness and is damaging to the brain and body.

> Everyone has some level of trauma to work on.

Trauma is so formidable because it means we have to deal with the aftermath of unwanted, unfair, and terrible experiences that are so hard to understand and process. Indeed, often the pain and confusion are so overwhelming that the protective instinct in our mind is to suppress them, which then affects our mental and brain health. In many cases, we will most likely never know the real *why* behind such an event; part of the healing process means getting comfortable with not having the *why* answered, which can make it so difficult to deal with. Rather than focusing so much time and mental energy on trying to find the *why*, it's much more helpful and healing to focus on using the 5 Steps to heal.

Remember, the mind works through the brain, and the brain responds to the mind. This means that suppressed trauma affects the brain and body. We saw this in our clinical trial: whatever happens in the nonconscious mind will be reflected in the brain. On a conscious level, we may think we have shoved it down far enough and even kid ourselves for a while that it has gone away, but this is not the case. The brain is not wired to handle toxic structures, and the nonconscious mind is all about balancing energy, so if we don't deal with our trauma, we can have breakdowns in our mind and/or body and brain, and these tend to be volcanic in nature due to their suppression.

Working on trauma includes little "t" traumas. Although these aren't pronounced traumatic events, they're damaging to our psyche and need attention. Some examples of this type of trauma can be interpersonal conflict, infidelity, legal troubles, or secondary trauma that results from indirect exposure to trauma through receiving a firsthand account or narrative of a traumatic event or helping a loved one who is going through trauma or suicidal ideation. Secondary trauma often produces *compassion fatigue*. First responders and health-care workers are at a great risk of secondary trauma, but family members, parents, and others can suffer as well. For example, you could be suffering secondary trauma if you were the one who helped get a sibling to the hospital after a suicide attempt. While you didn't experience the primary trauma, you did experience the secondary trauma—and your stressful experiences are also valid and need to be addressed.

Little "t" traumas are often overlooked because we rationalize them as common or not as serious or obvious as "big" traumas, so we don't deal with them. I want to stress that any type of trauma or adverse experience is something that needs to be addressed, *not* suppressed. Do not let shame or guilt keep you from healing.

When it comes to trauma, several factors are important: the impact, the cause, and the context, which work together. These are so important to deal with, because undealt-with trauma (all kinds) can become the filter through which you see the world and interact with others. The *impact* is how this filter is happening in your life in terms of how you see yourself and your relationships; the *cause* and the *context* work together and encompass what happened, your reaction to it, and how you managed it in order to cope at the time. These factors built a *thought pattern* and embedded memories into your brain, mind, and body. So, by first becoming aware of the impact (*embracing*), you can then find the cause and context (*processing*, mental autopsy), and then change this impact by reconfiguring (*reconceptualizing*). You do this using the 5 Steps.

When dealing with trauma recovery, I highly recommend working with a mental health professional or a trusted loved one, as it's helpful not to feel alone as you sort through intense emotions and thoughts. If you can't afford traditional therapy or aren't near any mental health professionals, there are plenty of amazing online therapy apps that work around the world 24/7 and offer very affordable plans. This doesn't mean neurocycling won't work for you; on the contrary, it will make your therapy more effective and give you the tools to cope between sessions on a day-to-day basis.

Here's what you do:

- Do the 5 Steps in seven- to thirty-minute time blocks, maximum, each day for twenty-one days. This is the mental autopsy, which will help you find and create the reconceptualized thought.

- Then, for the next forty-two days, spend five to seven minutes a day, spread across the day, *practicing* your newly reconceptualized thought.

- Work on just one thought for the whole 63-day cycle, which will help keep you focused. Remember, a thought is the big concept—the whole tree with all its branches, leaves, and roots. The branches and leaves are the memories (information and emotions) that your behaviors and communication come from; that is, what you're consciously thinking, saying, and doing. The tree trunk represents your perspective as experienced through the signals of happiness, joy, excitement, grief, depression, anxiety, and so on. The roots are the cause, or the origin story memories, which are made up of informational, emotional, and physical signals. There's a lot contained in one thought, which is why you stick with one at a time so you don't get overwhelmed.

- Follow the process: look at your behaviors first—the branches and leaves of the tree. Then look at the perspective attached to these behaviors—the tree trunk. Then track this to the origin story, the cause—the roots. You will get a little bit more insight each day. On day 1, you may see one behavior and emotion and kind of see the perspective, and by day 4 you may start seeing more behaviors and a clearer perspective and start glimpsing the origin. Just keep neurocycling forward over the twenty-one days.

- As you are working through this, all kinds of memories will surface, but don't let them overwhelm you. Capture them by briefly writing them down as you neurocycle. If they're associated with the current thought you're working on, then look at the insight they bring; if they are actually part of another thought, make a note to detox it during a later 63-day cycle. Don't forget to note these down somewhere, because they're from your nonconscious mind, and they're relevant in some way to your trauma.

To really make this work for you, you need to see neurocycling as a lifestyle, which means that as you finish one toxic trauma, you may want to take a little break for a short time and then work on the next trauma. Some traumas are really big and complicated and may take much longer to work through; others are not as big. The important thing to remember is that a suppressed trauma in the nonconscious mind can cause mental damage to your psyche and damage to your brain. But also remember: because of the power of your mind and neuroplasticity, this can all be healed.

I recommend keeping a journal to track what you decide to work and when. You're the only one who can make these decisions because only you really know what and how much you can handle. You may need to start talking to someone to work this out—a good therapist, coach, or counselor will know how to help you find this out for yourself, facilitating your healing journey. I also strongly recommend using my app with this book to work on trauma, as hearing and seeing someone walk you through this can be incredibly powerful.

Timing

As I mentioned above, dealing with trauma takes time. I recommend taking around seven to thirty minutes total per day for all of the 5 Steps, so around one and a half to five minutes per step. Trying to fix a trauma thought in one sitting will not work. You can also use the 5 Steps for trauma as a quick reminder, once you get the hang of neurocycling, if you find yourself triggered by something or someone.

Preparation

Begin each Neurocycle with a *calming and refocusing exercise.* This can be breathing, meditation, tapping, mindful meditation, prayer, Havening—whatever works for you. Doing this will align the mind-brain connection and facilitate the correct flow of delta, theta, alpha, beta, and gamma in the brain, which, in turn, optimizes the physiology and DNA of the cells of the body. As I said in the previous section, a lot of unseen and incredible brain, genetic, neuroendocrine, psychoneuroimmunological (mind-brain-immune system), and gut-brain things will happen in response. Over time, these repeated exercises will create neural networks (thought trees) that will be activated at will. I spend anywhere between thirty seconds and five to ten minutes in preparation, depending on what I'm dealing with.

Using the Neurocycle to Mind-Manage Trauma

Now, let's move on to applying the 5 Steps to trauma with another example from my own life.

1. **Gather.** Gather awareness of the emotional warning signal(s) and physical warning signal(s). Spend about two to five minutes on this step each day for twenty-one days. Be as clinical and analytical as you can be. To achieve this when working with trauma, use the following neuroplasticity practices (see chapter 9):

   - *Self-regulation.* When dealing with trauma, you may feel you have no control over your thoughts. But, actually, you do—you can learn to control them every ten seconds, to be precise. This means you can learn to be in control pretty much all the time.

   - *The Multiple Perspective Advantage.* This will help you distance yourself from the pain of your emotions.

   - *The 30–90 Second Rule.* It's never a good idea to react to any trigger immediately. That's especially true when it comes to trauma, because you're not in the optimal mind or brain state to respond in the thirty- to ninety-second adjustment period that will happen as you become aware of what's behind whatever you're working on.

     After my son was attacked in Rome, I started the healing process about three weeks later. Immediately after the event, I spent time and energy helping my son deal with his trauma. Each day I became a little more aware of each emotion and piece of information—the insight wasn't all there on day 1.

2. **Reflect.** Capture the thought and reflect on it. For example, by focusing on the hovering, nagging anxiety I had gathered awareness of, I realized I hadn't dealt with the actual

shock of my son being attacked, which had been written into my brain and body at the time of the incident and was at the back of my mind. Visualize grabbing the thought with your mind and getting a sense of the information. The MPA will help you separate the emotional, physical, and informational memories and control the emotional force that recalling trauma brings up. The limited time of three to five minutes also controls how much emotional exposure you have to the trauma, making it more digestible.

3. **Write.** Write everything from your reflections, no matter how jumbled—just get your mind and brain onto paper so you can really start seeing the mental mess and how to clean it up. Spend about five minutes on this each day. I wrote all my feelings and physical reactions onto my Metacog. Once I had done this, I started seeing how the traumas were separated in time and how each event had its own information, emotions, and physical reactions.

4. **Recheck.** This is the mental autopsy step, where we're figuring out how to "repair the brain" after doing our mental "surgery" in the previous steps. This also takes between three to five minutes daily for twenty-one days. One thing to really focus on in the Recheck step is forgiveness. Forgiveness is how you sever the tie with the person or persons who hurt you. How? Research shows that the details of a transgression, which can hold us in a viselike grip, are more susceptible to being reconceptualized and even forgotten when we forgive. Unforgiveness keeps the toxic thought tree strong and powerful in your brain, which impedes your healing because it's still "connected to the source." This is due to the law of entanglement in quantum physics, which keeps everything in a relationship—toxic or otherwise—entangled, affecting each component. When we forgive, we actually *grow* a part of our brain

called the anterior superior temporal sulcus (aSTS); the more we grow this area, the easier it will become to manage the pain of the trauma.[1]

I had to transfer the "pain energy" from what happened to "recovery energy," which is what I did with my Recheck step. I took the sting out of the story—it's still emotional, but it's *managed emotion*. This is where I started focusing on my reality: "My son survived, and he had no brain damage, even though he fell hard as they hit him repeatedly, which is a miracle. He has an amazing family, friends, and teachers who support him 24/7. We can speak and cry with pain but also joy. He went on to finish his study abroad and earned his degree with flying colors. He is helping others with trauma." I went from panicking and crying to having a possibilities mindset. I was guided by the *kintsugi* principle.

5. **Active Reach.** Speak the reconceptualized thought, saying it out loud—this will force you to focus on it and not the trauma. This takes only a few seconds to a couple of minutes, repeated throughout the day, so it is a really easy step to apply. Why do you need to do this? You want to remove energy from the thought; that is, stop watering the toxic thought tree so it "dies," transferring the energy to the healthy thought tree you are replacing it with. So, be very intentional about not allowing your mind to slip back into rehearsing the trauma. This will change the energy patterns of the brain, increasing the alpha-gamma pattern, which will make your mind stronger and more resilient. "Capture" the thought as it comes into your head, remembering that if you are conscious of something you can control it.

In my example, each time I found myself feeling physically sick rethinking about what happened to my son, I quickly captured the thought, acknowledged it, and replaced it with an Active Reach, which were statements like

"Jeff is alive and well! Remember the first hug as I saw him a few weeks later in Greece!" By doing this, I transferred the potential energy to go down a negative spiral to the truth of the current situation, and I did this with gratitude. This increased my cognitive resilience and directed my neuroplasticity, to the point that now I can tell you this story with controlled emotion—it's a terrifying story, but I'm in charge of it.

Four Helpful Techniques for Active Reaches to Process Trauma

As you progress forward in time through the shock of acute trauma—one hour later, one day later, and so on—here are four useful techniques you can practice as Active Reaches:

1. *Adopt a possibilities mindset.* Try to look for a few options or different ways of seeing the situation. There are so many possibilities a situation can end up resolving itself into. Even the worst situations have possibilities. In the midst of our family's crisis with my son, Jeffrey, we all kept saying things like "Maybe someone will have already helped him," "Maybe the police are there," *maybe, maybe, maybe.* We kept our hope active by imagining these possibilities. The next day we spoke to the program's professors about the possibility of improving the security training and briefings offered to study abroad students and teachers. Within a week new training protocols were implemented. One of the possibilities we saw came to fruition, and the program is now safer as a result. It bears repeating to mention that we tend to freeze up and lose cognitive flexibility in acute situations, which inevitably leads to poor decisions. A possibilities mindset really helps shift this "clog," but only if you practice it in easy times. You cannot just bandage an open

wound with positive statements. You have to believe that these possibilities actually exist, which takes time and work.

2. *Practice temporal distancing.* This basically means focusing on *the long term*, which will broaden your perspective and can help relieve emotional pressure in the moment. So, imagine you're an hour, a day, a week, or a year down the line. What does this situation look like? What's different? What have you learned? How have you changed? What

A Neurocycle Life Hack to End a Worry Spiral

Trauma that is not dealt with can lead to a worry spiral. If you have experienced something traumatic, such as a car accident, every time you get in a car you may find yourself worrying it may happen again; terrible events can shape how we see and interact with the world. This is part of the whole post-traumatic stress cycle, so here's a quick 5-Step hack to get the worry under control in the moment so you can focus on dealing with the root thought.

1. **Gather.** Gather awareness of what you are worrying about. Get into MPA mode as you look for the physical, emotional, and informational warning signals of your thoughts. As you observe the emotional and physical feelings from the worry, acknowledge them and start becoming aware of how you feel objectively, as if the emotions are in a box or behind a window in a building (see chapter 9).

2. **Reflect.** Imagine getting the emotional and informational memories of the worries out of your head and putting them into a box. The idea is to put the toxic worry into the box or window; you are on the outside looking in. You can't climb into the window or box—it's completely inaccessible—but you have power over whatever is in that window or box.

    Now, ask, answer, and discuss with yourself whether what you're worrying about will really happen. Is this worry based on fact or on advice would you give someone in a similar situation now that you've gained some hindsight? I did this when my son was attacked; I imagined meeting in Greece, as we were planning to do in a few weeks, and I hung on to that vision.

3. *Put the situation in a historical context.* Put acute stress in a historical context in terms of your own life (*I got through that terrible family situation several years ago; I can get through this*) or in general (*We got through the*

---

assumptions? What can you control in this situation? Can you make some kind of plan to work on this worry later on? In the past, has worrying about something ever actually helped the situation?

3. **Write.** Write the answers to your questions in a journal or on your smartphone or other device, or speak the answers to your questions out loud to yourself. Speaking back to yourself creates a temporary memory in the brain, which gives you a sense of control and helps organize your thoughts.

4. **Recheck.** Visualize the worst-case scenario very quickly, then move into solution mode: How would you handle it if it happened? What would your game plan be?

   Don't spend too long on this—just a few seconds. What steps would you take to solve the worst thing that could happen? Make sure you spend more time on solving than imagining the worst-case scenario, or you can end up making your worry worse!

   After you have done this, work back to what you would like the outcome to be. Give yourself a few scenarios as options, and have what I call a "possibilities mindset."

5. **Active Reach.** If you can, talk to someone to get perspective and clarity on what you worked out in the Recheck step. Type the possible solutions you worked out into your phone or other device, journal, or whatever works for you. You can then refer back to these as many times as you need if you feel the worry rising up again!

1918 Influenza, SARS, and MERS; we will get through COVID-19). The idea is to tell yourself that other people have gotten through times like these before, and so will you. You will get through this, maybe not unscathed, but you will come out the other side. This shifts your perspective and gives you hope.

4. *Think of a movie or show you have seen or book you have read that may remind you of your situation.* Sometimes this is as simple as a meme or statement that's comforting to you, which helps you process what you're facing.

No one can understand anyone else's trauma; you cannot be an expert on someone else's experience, no matter how many degrees you have. And no trauma should ever be judged or minimized. Our experiences should always be heard and validated and never labeled as a brain disease, which dehumanizes the person's experience. The brain will be impacted because the mind works through the brain, affecting its energy and blood flow, and this sets up a negative feedback loop between the mind and brain unless the memories are managed. I understand that suppression is a major survival mechanism, and that it can protect you and your mind in the moment, maybe even for a short time after, until you feel ready to cope. However, over the long term, suppression will wreak havoc in your mind, brain, and body. Granted, the hard work is scary, and it will take a lot of courageous effort to process and reconceptualize, but your mind is incredible—and so are you.

> *Dr. Leaf, I'm sure you get these messages all the time. I would be surprised if you didn't. I just want to honor you for your hard work. My mind is changing! I had a pretty significant traumatic experience in February of this year and have been reaching for a new perspective as a result. Choosing grace and forgiveness has brought so much peace. Thank you for leading people into hope and joy through your work! Love and thanks!*
>
> PETER

Chapter 13

Neurocycling to Break Bad Habits and Build Good Lifestyle Habits

It's not stress that kills us, it's our reaction to it.

Hans Selye

Overview

- If you're constantly stressed during the day, and you don't take the time to organize your thinking and reboot the brain, this can affect your sleeping patterns at night.

- When it comes to diet, there is no "one way" of eating. Each human being is unique. Throughout all my research, I have found only one overarching rule for eating: *eat real food mindfully.* When we understand the fundamentals of eating; that is, the completely entangled relationship between thinking and food and between our food and the world around us, we can make changes in our food choices.

- Exercise can improve all areas of cognitive function, including mood, thinking, learning, and memory, especially with age.

This chapter will cover using neurocycling to break bad habits and build good lifestyle habits. Bad habits include things like people-pleasing, poor sleeping patterns, an unhealthy diet, and lack of exercise. These bad habits and thinking patterns affect our mental and physical health.

Toxic Habits

Toxic habits are negative behavioral patterns we have established over time, like getting irritated in traffic, snapping at a loved one, or allowing ourselves to go down worry "rabbit holes" by always seeing the negative. Over time we build toxic habits into our mind and repeat them often, so we feel like they're a natural part of us. They really aren't, because we aren't wired for toxicity. They're destructive habits that can cause lots of toxic stress in our brains and bodies, as well as in relationships and life. They need to be identified, uprooted, and reconceptualized into constructive habits.

Using the Neurocycle to Mind-Manage Toxic Habits

A thought that's established is a thought that's gone through the cycle of being built into long-term memory and automatized over time, which happens over a period of around sixty-three days. Most of the time we aren't even consciously aware that we're building toxic thoughts into toxic habits—until we start acting on them on a regular basis and find they're affecting our mental health, physical health, and relationships.

In this section, I'm specifically referring to those toxic habits that irritate or worry us and those around us. These need to be dissected and examined with self-regulation—but you can do this only if you really want to change. You're the only one who can get you to that point of wanting to change and also the only one who can implement the change.

Here are some helpful tips to alert you to a toxic habit:

1. You repeatedly hear the same critique from those closest to you.
2. You find yourself needing to be extra defensive about a certain thing you did or said.
3. You resonate with an insecurity you've noticed in someone else and have tried to fix it in them.
4. As you develop your self-regulatory skills through using the 5 Steps, you become aware of toxic habits you have developed.
5. You notice a pattern of people reacting negatively to something you've said or done.
6. You notice a pattern as you start keeping a journal or thought diary.

No one likes to actively and intentionally seek out bad behaviors or habits because it goes against our self-protective instincts, yet if we don't, they'll only grow and make us feel worse mentally and physically. So, when you find yourself becoming defensive or trying to distract yourself from the awareness, *lean in to what you may be trying to avoid*. It will be ugly and messy, but if you don't address it, it will just stay ugly and messy.

Below is an example of how you could use the 5 Steps to deal with established toxic habits.

But First: Timing and Preparation

Dealing with toxic habits takes time, as we have discussed. And remember, always begin any 5-Step exercise with a *calming and refocusing exercise* that can be as short or as long as you want.

Belly breathing is easy to do and very relaxing. Try this basic exercise anytime you need to relax or relieve stress.

1. Sit or lie flat in a comfortable position.

2. Put one hand on your belly, just below your ribs, and the other hand on your chest.

3. Take a deep breath in through your nose and let your belly push your hand out. Your chest should not move.

4. Breathe out through pursed lips as if you were whistling. Feel the hand on your belly go in and use it to press all the air out.

5. Do this breathing three to ten times. Take your time with each breath.

6. Notice how you feel at the end of the exercise.

I also walk through other similar exercises in my Neurocycle app. Now, let's tackle a toxic habit with the 5 Steps.

1. **Gather.** Gather awareness of the impact that your general behavior has on others. Be brutally honest with yourself, because that's the only way you can start to change your habits. Remember, all toxic issues can be brain-damaging—no toxic habit is harmless.

   Is there a habit you have that may be irritating, upsetting, or disturbing a loved one, family member, or work colleague? Is there something you keep doing, something you don't want to do, that's affecting your mental health? Is it something you know you shouldn't be doing but keep doing anyway? What information, emotions, and physical warning signals are you sensing from your nonconscious mind when you think about this toxic habit, or as you become aware of it and notice you are upsetting others or yourself?

   For example, I personally had a really toxic habit for years of thinking, *If only I did it this way . . . If only I said that . . . I should have thought of this . . .* I would waste so much time in my head ruminating and imagining how things would've turned out so much better "if only." It stole my joy of the moment, and it impacted my relationship with my family. One day, my husband said to me that I needed to do a 21-day detox on my "if only" habit because it was frustrating everyone. I felt really bad at first, but I took his advice to follow my own advice, and I did it. I did the 5 Steps over sixty-three days—and was stunned at how much my toxic habit had affected my joy and inner peace. Once you gather awareness, it's very hard to want to go back to bad habits.

2. **Reflect.** Reflect on this habit by using the Multiple Perspective Advantage (MPA) practice. Stand back and observe yourself, which will help separate you from what you are doing. This will prevent you from getting stuck in shame, condemnation, or victimization, which can happen when we face the toxic habits we have developed over time.

   Do you think your toxic habit is the common denominator that messes up your relationships? What effect is this having on you? Do you see the need to change it? Why? Are there triggers? Is it irritating, upsetting, or disturbing others? Is there something you keep doing that is affecting your mental health, something you know you shouldn't be doing but keep doing anyway?

   Using my "if only" example, I hadn't realized that I was doing this so often and was being tormented by it and letting it waste my time. It took me a full twenty-one days of doing the 5 Steps daily to be able to admit this habit to myself and see what it was doing. Do you have more than one bad habit? (Generally, we do.) Prioritize your toxic habits and select the most dominant one to work on first.

3. **Write.** Write your answers to the above questions. It doesn't matter how disorganized this writing is, just get the information out of your mind and brain and onto paper. For example, if more than one toxic habit popped up, you can quickly write down a brief list somewhere if you want to work on something later on. This is where the Metacog is so useful (see *Think, Learn, Succeed* for more information on the Metacog).

   In my example, writing helped me see deeper into my thinking patterns and gain insight into my mind. Using the Metacog helped me really integrate the impact of my "if only" behavior and see what it was doing to me and my family.

4. **Recheck.** Look at what you have written. Think about what you can do instead of the toxic habit. This is a mental autopsy, so pull your toxic habit apart mentally and see how you can change your behavior. Can you trace it back to its origin? In my "if only" example, over the twenty-one days I saw that I had a strong desire to never be wrong and for everything to be perfect all the time, and this was giving me a false sense of value and worth.

   Now, use the emotional warning signal guide on page 204 to rate the intensity of the emotion you are feeling and see how much it has changed from Gather to Recheck. This should just take a couple of seconds. Use this step to find triggers, patterns, common themes, maybe even common reactions.

5. **Active Reach.** Design an Active Reach, completing these three statements:

   My physical trigger is _____

   My reconceptualized information is _____

   My reconceptualized feelings are _____

Now, create an Active Reach that fills in these three blanks:

*When I experience the physical trigger of _____,
I will tell myself _____ and choose
to feel _____.*

Or your Active Reach could be even simpler, like:

*When I start to feel _____, I am going to do the
belly breathing technique.*

Remind yourself to work on wiring the new, healthy, reconceptualized habit into your brain over the next sixty-three days by adding it to the reminders on your phone, the reminders on your Neurocycle app, a sticky note on the fridge, or whatever works for you. Each time it pops up will be a conscious reminder to practice the new thought habit. As you're doing this, you'll likely come across other toxic habits along the way, so add them to your list and work on them after the first one is sorted out.

In my "if only" example above, I realized I needed to adopt a thinker mindset, which would allow me to accept and appreciate the moment for what it was and reconceptualize the "if only" thoughts into possibilities for the future as opposed to failures in the moment. So, my Active Reaches were statements like "It's okay to analyze what I did wrong in this situation, but only if I take hold of the lesson—what's the lesson here?" and "Remember not to see if-onlys as negatives of what I didn't do but possibilities of what I can do in the future." This set me free from the anxiety and loss of joy I was experiencing on a daily basis. Another Active Reach phrase I used that helped me—and still does, when I catch myself in a potentially negative if-only moment—is "I cannot change the past, but I can learn from it and improve my present and future."

I personally spent about seven minutes each day working through the 5 Steps for the first twenty-one days, and then a few seconds to read and use my final Active Reach: "Remember, no if-onlys today!" about seven times a day for the next forty-two days. These forty-two days went by very quickly, even though I kept working on my "if only" habit by keeping it in the forefront of my conscious mind to practice it, giving it enough energy to live in the nonconscious mind and impact my behavior. I was changing the neuroplasticity of my brain with each little step, right down to the quantum vibrations in the tubulin of the microtubules of my dendrites!

Small changes are very effective over time, and they have a cumulative impact on our behavior. Using your reminders daily until you hit day 63 may seem cumbersome at times, but it means you are conquering that toxic habit and building the new, reconceptualized, and healthy way of thinking! During this process, you will be very cognizant of your toxic habit throughout the first twenty-one days as it becomes a long-term memory; thereafter it will become easier and easier to work on.

This is something you will be able to pull on automatically when you need it. For instance, now when I get the emotional warning signal of hovering anxiety and physical warning signal of a cramped stomach after something has happened, I pay attention. Through the 5 Steps over the 63-day cycle, I'd observed that these two warning signals went hand in hand with my "if only" issue, which does creep back from time to time—and this is completely normal! However, now I know what to do to beat it; it no longer controls me. I control all my "if only's," including their ugly cousins "would have," "should have," and "could have."

Managing Human Connection

Human beings are made for connection. We aren't meant to do life alone. Whether we are a so-called introvert or extrovert, we need community. We function at our best in groups of people where we enhance, not just compete with, one another. To quote Mother

A Neurocycle Life Hack to Mind-Manage the Habit of People-Pleasing

Here's another example of how to use neurocycling for a common toxic habit: people-pleasing.

1. **Gather**. Gather awareness about times you've noticed yourself people-pleasing and any emotions and physical sensations associated with these memories. What did you think and feel then? What do you think and feel now?

2. **Reflect.** Now ask yourself questions like:
   Why did I say yes in that moment when I wanted to say no?
   What happened when I said yes? How did I feel? Was it helpful or harmful to me?
   When do I tend to do the most people-pleasing? What scenario, situation, or environment?
   Who do I try to please the most? Why?
   What if I said no? Why am I afraid to say no?
   Am I trying to hide an insecurity?
   Am I afraid of being alone?

3. **Write.** Write down your thinking and your answers to the questions above. Are there triggers? Patterns? Can you take some of your questions and answers deeper? How will you reconceptualize this and reconfigure what you will do and say in a way that moves you away from people-pleasing?

4. **Recheck.** Go back over what you wrote. Are there triggers? Patterns? Can you take some of your questions and answers deeper? How can you reconceptualize this and reconfigure what you will do and say in a way that moves you away from people-pleasing?

5. **Active Reach.** Often people tend to people-please as a coping strategy for dealing with loneliness or even with self-confidence issues. If you find a lack of self-confidence is an issue for you, your Active Reach can be something as simple as spending more time on using the 5 Steps to boost your self-esteem, like identity and brain-building, or you could even set a reminder to intentionally notice how many times during the day you say yes or do something for someone that you do not want to do.

A Neurocycle Life Hack to Mind-Manage the Habit of Toxic Ruminating

Ruminating gets you stuck in the hamster wheel of going around and around with no progression forward and can really challenge your value and identity and make you feel useless.

1. **Gather** awareness of past times you have ruminated and caught yourself overthinking. What physical and mental warning signals did you notice? What do you feel now mentally and physically?

2. **Reflect.** Ask yourself, *Why did I feel this way? What triggered this overthinking moment? What content was I overthinking? Were (are) my thoughts based on fact or assumption? How do I respond to overthinking?*

3. **Write.** Make a Metacog if you have time, or if not, visualize making one, because this writes it genetically in the brain.

4. **Recheck:** Do you notice any triggers or patterns? Can you go deeper with some questions and answers? What assumptions do you notice?

5. **Active Reach.** Remind yourself that when you start to notice you're overthinking, you will immediately do something physical like run a few sprints or dance. Or educate yourself on the difference between overthinking and thinking deeply.

Teresa, "I can do things you cannot, you can do things I cannot: together we can do great things."[1]

There is endless research showing that engaging positively with a social support network, in a giving as well as a getting way, correlates with a number of desirable outcomes. Being part of a community helps us clean up the mental mess with improved cognitive resilience, a reduction in chronic pain, lower blood pressure, and improved cardiovascular health.[2] When we engage with others, our cortisol levels go down while the neurotransmitters serotonin and dopamine balance in our brains. We have higher levels of all the brain waves that promote healing and lower levels of anxiety-linked high beta. We feel good subjectively, and this translates into changes in our cells. Mind becomes matter as our brains are flooded with pleasure-inducing endorphins, intimacy-producing oxytocin, and the bliss molecule anandamide.

Just think about the last time you felt really sad and a friend or family member came and sat with you or reached out and just supported you. It didn't make the situation you were sad about go away, but it did help you feel better and more able to face the problem.

Today we are more connected, thanks to amazing innovations in technology, yet feel more disconnected socially than ever before. Technology is not going away, so we need to focus our energy on managing it to our advantage—and managing our minds so we are not being taken advantage of. Remember, it's not about the number of connections you have; it is about the quality of your connections. Here are some simple and quick ways to improve the quality of your connections and fight loneliness:

1. Join a fitness studio that offers group classes.
2. Volunteer at a church, community center, or local nonprofit.
3. See a therapist or other mental health professional.
4. Invest in current relationships by letting those close to you know how much you appreciate them, take an interest in what they are interested in (even if it sounds boring to you!), write them a letter letting them know how much they mean to you, call them, or when spending time together put away devices and listen.
5. Join a club or start a club.

Accept that loneliness isn't something to be ashamed of or brushed aside because it seems silly. First of all, question where those notions are coming from—is it some form of toxic masculinity, pride, or cultural influence? Second, if you suppress even minor feelings they will get worse. It may seem like you're being strong by "going it alone" but I can promise you this approach is counterproductive and will damage your mental and physical health.

We also need to shift our mindset to celebrating and enhancing others rather than competing with them. Do you have a zero-sum mindset where you think if someone wins, someone else must lose? This mindset is very toxic and will not only ruin relationships but also decrease your ability to heal.

When you feel more connected and happy, you can support, notice, and listen to others. This will not only help them but you as well—people who help others can experience up to a 68 percent increase in their own healing![3] Additionally, research from Berkeley, California, shows that focusing on doing things for others in the sense of being part of a community will increase your joy and happiness versus focusing just on yourself,[4] while another recent study found that social support was the greatest predictor of happiness during periods of high stress.[5]

How to Use the Neurocycle to Develop Better Connection Habits

1. **Gather.** Gather awareness of your emotional, physical, and informational warning signals. Are you feeling lonely? Does being alone make you feel sick? Do your worst mental health moments happen when you are alone, or when you are with others but they are so disconnected from you or undervalue you so much as a person that you feel alone? Also gather awareness of how much you are actually reaching out and engaging with others in your community.

2. **Reflect.** Reflect on why you feel like this. Why are or aren't you reaching out to others, and if you are, how? Is it working? Where are the gaps in not just being you but *being you in the world*? When you want to feel happy, do you do things for yourself or for others? When have you been happiest in your life? Who were you with in these moments? Are you avoiding connections because you feel like you are not good enough? Do you feel you need to always be "on" when around people? Why? Could people-pleasing be keeping you from deep, meaningful connections?

3. **Write.** Write down your answers from the Reflect step. Be honest with yourself and be vulnerable.

4. **Recheck.** Reconceptualize, redesign, and change your perception. How can you listen more to others? How can you reach out and be a part of your community? Can you help someone financially, with food, or with child care?

   Look around the world and see how communities function. Think of ways you can make a difference in your community. Can you introduce deep discussions with interesting people that challenge you to really go beyond yourself? How can you make community engagement a lifestyle? What patterns are you noticing?

5. **Active Reach.** Choose one or two of the answers you wrote in the Recheck step and do it today. Keep doing this or something new to connect with others in some meaningful way each day, even if it's as simple as texting someone that you are thinking about them! In sixty-three days this will become a lifestyle habit that can improve your well-being, peace, and happiness. Indeed, in my clinical practice I always included an aspect of helping someone else as part of any treatment; this is the principle of "get a session, give a session."

Here are a few more community Active Reaches you can do: when you feel burdened with work, are emotionally challenged, or are going through something, try stopping for a moment and helping someone else, even if it's just to listen, hug, or encourage them. Send an email or text telling them you are thinking of them, or invite someone to lunch or dinner instead of eating alone. When you are in a small space with a stranger, like an elevator, smile and say hello instead of looking at the floor or your phone. My husband, Mac, does this every time, and it amazes me that by the time we get to our floor, he already knows their life history and has a new friend!

Better Sleep Habits

We all know sleep is really important. However, research also suggests there's a huge cost to pathologizing it. This means that worrying about sleep and identifying and labeling yourself as a poor sleeper may be worse than not sleeping.

There's endless research telling us the impact of sleep deprivation and that sleep serves a myriad of functions. Personally, when someone tells me "You need to sleep or you will be too tired for whatever tomorrow brings," or "Go to sleep early so you don't damage your brain," I won't sleep just because I start panicking about not sleeping! It also doesn't always help that everyone in the wellness/medical space keeps saying, "Sleep or else." It's like pouring fuel on the fire of your panic, which makes everything worse.

I have been there many times. I have done almost everything when I cannot sleep: counting sheep, deep 4–7–8 breathing, a hot bath ninety minutes before bedtime, switching off my cell phone two hours before bedtime, exercising at night and in the morning, removing the TV from my bedroom, avoiding work before bed, reading a book in bed, taking melatonin, drinking chamomile tea

. . . I have even tried to convince myself I was asleep, and I still stayed awake trying not to worry about being awake!

As a scientist, I could write a whole book about sleep deprivation—and I would probably only make you a worse sleeper. I am not going to do that. I want to help you think differently about sleep. Sometimes poor sleep is inevitable, and that's not necessarily a catastrophe. We have the ability to handle sleepless nights now and then, and some people genetically just need less sleep.[6] It's also better to focus on how many sleep cycles you have in a week versus sleep hours in a night.

The good news is that every version of the 5 Steps for mind-management in part 2 is a kind of sleep prep, so if you do any of these, you're already preparing your mind, brain, and body for better sleep.

Using the Neurocycle for AM Sleep Prep

1. **Gather.** Preparing for sleep begins in the morning, as counterintuitive as this may sound. The way your mind is managed from the time you wake up impacts the biochemistry, circadian rhythm, and energy of the brain. An unmanaged, messy mind is an unmanaged, messy brain that will result in messy sleep. Gather awareness of your thinking. What is going through your mind? Are you anxious about something? How do you feel physically? Do you still feel tired? Did you wake up in a panic? What did you dream? Do this as soon as you wake up, before you get on your phone. I find it helpful to do this Gather step as part of my morning meditation.

2. **Reflect.** Reflect on what you're focusing on as you wake up. Is it on the problems and negative aspects of the day or the bits and pieces of your dreams, images from TV, and undealt-with thoughts flowing messily and chaotically in your mind? What is occupying your attention? Are you

anxious? What are you excited about today? What are you dreading?

3. **Write.** If you don't catch your thoughts with their intertwined emotions, information, and embodied physical sensations, this messy waking up state can become a messy day, and you will feel like you are playing catch-up all day. So, *think*; say your thoughts out loud or write them quickly into your journal next to your bed.

4. **Recheck.** Recheck your thoughts by breathing in for three counts and out for three counts, saying the opposite of what you captured; for example, "I can only try to do what I can, and it's fine if I don't finish," instead of "I have so much to do today!"

5. **Active Reach.** Choose to put on a mindset for the day. For more on mindsets, see my book *Think, Learn, Succeed*. Here are some more helpful morning Active Reach reminders:

   1. Write five things you are proud of yourself for—start your day off celebrating yourself!

   2. Write five things you are grateful for.

   3. Ask yourself not what you want to or have to *do* today but rather who you want to *be* today and how you want to feel.

   4. Set reminders or write a note to remind yourself that no matter what happens today, it will be a great day.

   5. Ask yourself these three questions: *What am I letting go of? What am I grateful for? What am I focusing on?*

Using the Neurocycle for During the Day Sleep Prep

If you're constantly stressed during the day, and you don't take the time to organize your thinking and reboot the brain, this can affect your sleeping patterns at night. When you go to sleep, you're going into a "housekeeping" mode—everything is getting cleaned up, which helps prepare you for the next day. If there's a lot of mental mess in the brain, this housekeeping function is hindered, which can affect how you sleep (including nightmares) and how you feel the next day.

Many of us tend to panic at night as we're trying to go to sleep, because our brains are exhausted from chaotic thinking patterns during the day. That's why it is so important to take thinker moments throughout the day when we switch off to the external and switch on to the internal, and just let our minds wander. These moments give your brain a rest and allow it to reboot and heal, which increases your clarity of thought and organizes the networks of your brain by balancing alpha and beta activity. This increases blood flow to the brain, which helps it function better and helps you deal with challenges and stress.

The opposite will happen if you don't take regular thinker moments. Not giving the mind a rest can reduce blood flow by up to 80 percent in the front of the brain, which can dramatically affect cognitive fluency and the efficient, associative thinking required at school or in the workplace. Cumulatively, this can lead to unprocessed thoughts and constant nightmares, affecting overall quality of sleep and performance.

Thinker moments can be anything from a short ten seconds to a full hour. If possible, I highly recommend going outside while doing them. The vitamin D from the sunshine and the fresh air will greatly improve your mood and physical health. To do a thinker moment, simply close your eyes and let your mind wander. Daydream, listen to some music, take a walk, even doodle. You will be surprised to notice what thoughts and feelings pop up from your nonconscious during these moments. Take note of them and then plan on addressing them using the 5 Steps. I sometimes just stop and stare out a window for a few seconds, and I find this very helpful and invigorating. Research shows that thinker moments actually increase our intelligence and efficiency, and therefore help clean up the mental mess in preparation for sleep.

Using the Neurocycle for PM Sleep Prep

1. **Gather.** Gather awareness of your mental space before bed. Is it messy? Tidy? Sort of organized? How are you feeling mentally and physically? What moments of your day stand out to you? How was the overall quality of your day? What did you learn today? Did anything about your day make you especially happy, sad, or anxious?

2. **Reflect.** Reflect on the information and emotions of these thoughts as you get ready for bed. Remember, you control what you want to think about; you control your neuroplasticity. What do you want in your head before you go to sleep? The thoughts you take to bed will affect the regeneration and preparation processes that occur at night.

   It's not important to solve everything before you go to bed, but it is important to acknowledge what is nagging at you and then plan how you'll solve it—don't just leave the thoughts hanging, and don't suppress them. This causes cognitive dissonance, which can lead to disturbing dreams and make you feel really bad the next day. The key is to get it all out and plan to resolve it.

   It's vital to realize that unmanaged thoughts will create chaotic, toxic energy in the brain, which can keep you awake at night, causing brain damage and mental health issues. Chaotic, toxic thoughts create a mental mess and need to be embraced, acknowledged, isolated, and compartmentalized in order to be processed and reconceptualized in a healthy fashion. They should never be ignored or suppressed, as I have said throughout this book.

You can do this proactively by getting into a regular mind detox routine. Just seven to fifteen minutes a day of detoxing your mind can improve your sleeping patterns—you are cleaning up your mental mess and getting your mind right before bed, which helps your brain and body regenerate at night. If deep-seated issues are keeping you awake at night, you can do a 21-day detox (see chapter 10) and use my SWITCH app to help overcome this.

3. **Writing.** Writing is a great way to prepare for sleep. It's like sweeping up a mess in your mind: you know the dirt will come again, but for now you can enjoy a clean floor. Writing helps you pour your brain on paper, getting it out into the conscious mind where you can start making sense of it.

   Write your reflections from step 2, and, as you do this, visualize a little vacuum cleaning your brain and allowing the necessary neurochemicals to flow like they should in preparation for sleep. Then, in deep sleep, the nonconscious mind can consolidate the thoughts and integrate them, and when you wake up, prompt you in the right direction. "Sleeping on it" really is very scientific.

4. **Recheck.** Recheck what you have written by writing a short, simple statement like, "I know this issue is huge, but I know I will find a solution. I don't have to find it now, and worrying now will only make it worse." Now, simply read over what you have written. Do you see a pattern in your thinking that emerged a few times during the day? How did that thinking affect your work or interactions? Did you take enough thinker moments? If you did have a fight with someone or a stressful moment, what were the triggers?

5. **Active Reach.** Your nighttime Active Reach could be writing a list of what you *did do* today versus what you *didn't do*. This is an excellent way to calm down your nervous

system to help you sleep. For example: "I maximized my time today," "I chose to rest and do nothing, which was great for the brain," "I did some exercise, and tomorrow I will add five more minutes," "I ate well today—some really great real food," or "I spent time with my family."

If you find yourself unable to sleep, don't allow yourself to lie in bed panicking about not sleeping. Instead, get excited and embrace the fact you're awake. Tell yourself, *This is going to be a nice, quiet time, where I'm not bugged by texts, emails, or people needing something. I am going to get that research done, finally read that book, watch that program on the Discovery Channel, tidy that closet, or work uninterrupted on a project!*

That excitement lowers your cortisol levels, balances the HPA axis (the "stress axis"), and makes stress work for you and not against you, activating your resilience and changing your genes in a good way. So, when you can't sleep, develop a positive expectation mindset that this is a special time just for you that you'll use wisely. This will help you get your panic under control and improve your well-being. However, a negative expectation mindset, where you imagine all the things that can go wrong if you don't sleep, is just going to damage your brain and make you feel worse—it's not worth it!

Another great Active Reach tip is to not let that adrenaline keep pumping. If you get into bed at night, fall asleep, and then wake up with a "whoosh" of adrenaline, don't lie there marinating in this potentially damaging energy. Instead, sit up immediately, open your eyes, breathe deeply (in for four counts, hold for seven counts, and out for eight counts), and start shifting your energy in the right direction. Use the energy from the adrenaline; it has reset your brain and body to be alert, not sleepy, and fighting it sends conflicting messages to your brain and will make your attempt to sleep worse.

Reconceptualize the situation into something positive and do something constructive, because lying there just trying to sleep is not helpful. Write down whatever is on your mind—just pour it out. If it's a bunch of worries, plan to work on them as you do your daily detox. If it's a list of things to do, write them down and work out when you are going to do them, how long it will take, and who is going to help you. Pray or meditate over them if you wish. Tell yourself you will deal with them tomorrow. Choose to be excited and expectant that solutions will come and, no matter what they are, you will be at peace! This generates a flow of healthy, healing energy through your brain and can help you fall asleep.

Better Food Habits

When it comes to diet, there's no one way of eating. Each human being is unique. Throughout all my research, I've found only one overarching rule for eating: *eat real food mindfully.* When we understand the fundamentals of eating, the completely entangled relationship between thinking and food and between our food and the world around us, we can make changes in our food choices. I understand that, like exercise, there is so much advice out there on what to eat and what not to eat that it can be incredibly confusing. Having one overarching rule can make it a lot easier to change our diet and establish nourishing eating habits in the best possible way we can.

When I say "real food," what do I mean? What else can we eat? Unfortunately, this is where our current industrial food system has tricked us. Despite the apparent diversity of foodstuffs in our grocery stores, restaurants, and homes, many of the products available for purchase today are industrially manufactured "food-like products."[7] They contain unfamiliar substances that extend shelf life and flavor, and are often derived from just three highly processed commodities: corn, soy, and wheat. Real food, on the other hand, is fresh and nutritious, predominantly local, seasonal, grass-fed, as wild as possible, free of synthetic chemicals, whole or minimally processed, and ecologically diverse. When we care about the way our food is produced and care about "what the animals we eat, eat," we consume foods that are the most nourishing for us.[8]

Like everything in life, we cannot change our eating habits until we fully comprehend what needs to be changed. Your mind drives the effective functioning of your digestive system; if you eat with a messy mind, you will have a messy stomach and GI tract! Eating without cleaning up the mental mess means your mind will impact your digestive system, and vice versa. I always used to tell my patients that if you think right, you will eat right, and if you eat right, you will think right. There is plenty of research out there on the relationship between psychological stress and metabolic stress, so it's important to work on these together as opposed to individually, as they are often interdependent.[9] (For more information on eating, and how to make real food available to everyone, please see my book *Think and Eat Yourself Smart*, where I explore eating real food mindfully in depth.)

As you use the 5 Steps below, be gracious with yourself, because changing your food choices can be difficult, but as soon as you get your head around it, it becomes much easier.

Using the Neurocycle to Mind-Manage Better Food Habits

1. **Gather.** Gather awareness of what you're eating today and what you generally eat during a week. How do you feel mentally and physically when you eat or when you shop for groceries?

2. **Reflect.** Reflect on specific food items, meals, and ingredients in your fridge, pantry, and shopping list—are you eating *real food*? Do you eat when you are stressed, angry, or upset? How does this make you feel? Do you want to eat real food? What are your reasons for choosing the food you do? How can you slowly introduce more real foods into your lifestyle?

   You can also ask yourself questions like:

   What is my relationship with food? Is it healthy?

   How do I feel after eating?

   Why do I feel the need to count calories?

   Why do certain foods or meals trigger me?

   *Do I put enough or too much attention on food and
      eating?*

3. **Write.** Write down your current food choices, as well as the answers to your questions in step 2. It may be helpful to keep a food diary where you not only write down what you ate, when, and how but also how you felt mentally and physically before and after eating.

4. **Recheck.** Do you notice any patterns? Common themes or triggers? Can you go further with certain questions and answers from step 2? Ask yourself questions about what you wrote down. Some good questions are, *What do I eat and why? Where do I buy my food? Do I eat when I am stressed, angry, or upset? What is my "eating mood"? Do I ever "cheat"? How do I understand "cheating"? What foods should I try to avoid? What foods do I eat a lot of? How do I cook my food? What am I teaching my children about food and eating?*

5. **Active Reach.** Take action today, but start small: How can you change one meal today, making it a "real food mindfully" meal? Or perhaps you can go to your pantry

or fridge and get rid of one or more "food-like products." Think of ways you can start making small changes to how you think about and how you eat food.

Keep repeating steps 1 through 5 as you develop and grow your eating plan over the next sixty-three days. Before you know it, you will be well on your way to eating real food mindfully and feeling better! Write these five basic steps as a reminder wherever you will see them often. Remember, *you control* your food choices.

Better Exercise and Movement Habits

Exercise can improve all areas of cognitive function, including thinking, learning, and memory, especially with age. Most explanations we hear for why exercise makes us happy are too simplistic—it's not just an endorphin rush. Movement of any kind influences your whole biochemistry and brain energy, giving you hope and energy and helping to alleviate worry, even assisting with bonding. It reduces inflammation in the brain, which over time can protect against depression, anxiety, and loneliness. During exercise, muscles secrete hormones into our bloodstream that scientists are calling "hope chemicals!"[10]

In children, exercise is incredibly important for memory development. And the older you get, the more you need to move on a daily basis, even if it is in short bursts or power walking up those stairs instead of using the elevator. Indeed, our overall ability to think and understand is improved with exercise, regardless of our age. Physical activity increases blood flow to the anterior cingulate cortex (deep inside the middle of the brain), which is activated when we shift between thoughts in a flexible manner.

Not only are we better able to form memories when we move but we also improve communication between these memories, facilitating deep and meaningful understanding. Adding to these benefits, certain hormones that increase during exercise help improve memory and thinking. These hormones are growth factors called brain-derived neurotrophic factor (BDNF), vascular endothelial growth factor (VEGF), and insulin-like growth factor 1 (IGF-1).[11] In fact, people who exercise often improve their memory performance and show greater increase in brain blood flow to the hippocampus, the key brain region that deals with converting short- to long-term memory and is particularly affected by Alzheimer's disease.[12] In short, your brain loves exercise!

Physical activity also changes our DNA for the better. The epigenetic pattern of genes that affect fat storage in the body actually changes with exercise—the more we move, the better our bodies get at using and storing fat. Methyl groups on genes can be influenced in various ways through exercise, diet, and lifestyle, in a process known as *DNA methylation*. Researchers have found that when we exercise, epigenetic changes occur in seven thousand of the twenty thousand to twenty-five thousand genes, with positive changes in genes linked to type 2 diabetes and obesity![13]

Other studies have shown that when we exercise, our body almost immediately experiences genetic activation that increases the production of fat-busting proteins.[14] So thinking well, eating well, and physical exercise are therefore necessary to maintaining a healthy body weight and lifestyle. Although exercise fads come and go, the main thing to remember is to move as much as possible! Find out what works well for your body type and maintain a routine, one that suits your schedule and abilities.

The many benefits of movement are not limited to physical health. Research has shown that people who are more physically active are happier, have more meaningful lives, have better relationships, experience more positive emotions, deal with depression and anxiety better, and have more hope—all these increase longevity.[15] Every time we move our body, we are giving ourselves a dose of happiness and health and are investing in our mental health.

Exercise is one of the best ways to boost your mood; it releases the body's natural antidepressants and anxiolytics (with no side effects) and comes with a deep sense of peace and satisfaction.

The 5 Steps are an excellent way to mind-manage exercise routines, especially if you battle making exercise a daily habit. There are so many fun and joyful ways you can start incorporating exercise into your life. All movement is good movement!

Using the Neurocycle to Mind-Manage Healthy Exercise

1. **Gather.** Gather awareness of what exercise and movement you *are* or *aren't* doing. How do you feel mentally and physically before and after movement? When do you have your best or worst workouts? What are your general attitude and feelings toward movement and exercise?

2. **Reflect.** Ask yourself questions like:

   Why do I avoid working out?

   Do I use exercise as a distraction or way of trying to bring control to my life?

   Why do I feel how I feel before or after a workout?

   What could I do to make movement a more sustainable habit in my life?

   What information about exercise and working out could I use as motivation?

   Use your answers to make a list of benefit statements for exercise. Think of what movement you love and see how you can fit this into your day. What simple activity could you do right now?

   One note to keep in mind: exercise is simply movement. Don't let yourself get caught up in the idea that you have to run on a treadmill for an hour to get your "exercise" points. Simply going for a walk or cleaning your house is a great form of exercise! I personally love taking long walks and listening to insightful and interesting podcasts, which not only helps build my brain but also strengthens my physical body.

3. **Write.** Write this all down in an exercise journal. Take note of the types of workouts and times so you can start to find what works best for you. Intentionally noting information like this will help you determine a manageable and enjoyable plan of action that will lead to sustainable growth and change. Simply going through life without intentionally noting thoughts, feelings, actions, and reactions will not help you when trying to break or build a habit.

4. **Recheck.** Recheck to see what you can add if you do have an exercise routine, or what you can start with if you don't have one. What are your motivations for working out? Is there room for improvement? How does exercise make you feel? How can you keep up the momentum? What patterns are you noticing?

   Check your thoughts as you exercise, because toxic thoughts can reduce the antidepressant and anxiolytic effects of movement, so throw yourself into exercise with a good attitude and watch your mood improve.

5. **Active Reach.** Now, move! Take action today—don't put it off until tomorrow or next week or next month. It'll never happen unless you start where you are. And reward your effort with how you feel afterward (not junk food!).

   Some Active Reach ideas:

   1. Go into exercise with a thought like, *This is good for me and will help calm me down and make me feel better mentally and physically. This is another tool I am using to clean up my mental mess.*

   2. Plan the what, when, and how of your exercise routine for today. A short ten- to fifteen-minute walk? Maybe a five-minute workout video on YouTube? Five sprints

in your local park or driveway? Some Zumba dancing, then a walk with the dog?

3. Try a different workout routine or class for the next twenty-one days to find what you like and do not like.

4. Take a walk every day for the next twenty-one days.

5. During your day, take short two- to five-minute workout breaks. I love doing a few ab exercises, or sometimes I even just run up and down my stairs!

I have completed the 5 Steps. In the beginning it was very overwhelming, but in the end it was amazing to have reconceptualized the toxic thoughts. Fear . . . will no longer hold me back. Thank you so much; this is a beginning to a new lifelong lifestyle change for good. The next cycle I want to do with a friend. Many thanks.

TRACEY

Chapter 14

Neurocycling as a Daily Mind-Management Routine for Cleaning Up the Mental Mess

*Peace of mind is attained not by ignoring
problems but by solving them.*

RAYMOND HULL

Overview

- When we wake up in the morning, our first priority should be to get our mind into the right mental space for the day, not to catch up on social media or see what is happening on the news. How we spend the first few minutes of the day is incredibly important, because it can set the tone for the rest of the day.

- Brain-building is a great way to calm down, especially if you have just had a bad argument or are in a toxic situation. It restabilizes brain energy and chemicals, which often feel like they have been put in a blender when arguments and toxic things happen to us.

> • How you use your mind to manage your mind is so incredibly important. It is the foundation of a happy and healthy life because it helps you make the choices that lead to a happy and healthy life.

So, all this sounds great but . . . how do all these tips and techniques work in real life? What could mind-management look like in *your* life?

In this last chapter, I'll show you what my daily "cleaning up the mental mess" routine looks like and how I have developed this into a mind-management lifestyle. I've designed my daily routine to optimize mind, body, and brain function, and help facilitate all the wonderful benefits I've been telling you about throughout this book. I'm hoping my examples will help you find and develop your own daily mind-management routine that works best for you. If you wish, you can take this and the information in the previous chapters and adapt them to your lifestyle.

There are eight parts to this daily process:

1. Getting my mind ready for the day (thirty seconds to two minutes).

2. Brain-building (fifteen to sixty minutes—more if I have time, because the more deep thinking I do, the better).

3. Trauma and habit detoxing using the Neurocycle (seven to fifteen minutes). I alternate between a trauma detox and a habit detox every sixty-three days.

4. Thinker moments (five seconds to a couple of minutes every hour, when tired, plus ten minutes early morning or midday, in the sun if possible).

5. Active Reach seven times throughout the day (one to three minutes). I use the reminder function on my app to do this.

6. Listening to my body and eating real food mindfully, including three to five fasted workouts a week.

7. Moving my body (sixty to eighty minutes of exercise daily, moving around, and sixty to ninety minutes of thermal exercise in an infrared sauna).

8. I use AM, daytime, and PM neurocycling for my sleep routine throughout the day.

1. Getting My Mind Ready for the Day

As soon as I wake up, I start getting my mind ready for the day. This takes around thirty seconds to two minutes. My objective is to give my biochemistry and brain energy a chance to settle so I can get the best out of my brain throughout the day.

When we wake up in the morning, our first priority should be to get our mind into the right mental space for the day, not to catch up on social media or see what is happening on the news. How we spend the first few minutes of the day is incredibly important, because it can set the tone for the rest of the day. Why? When we wake up, our mind is swirling with energy and our attention is scattered and dysfunctional. It's so easy in this state to let our focus drift to our problems, the negative aspects of the day coming up, unresolved issues from yesterday, bits and pieces of our dreams, or what is happening in the world—all the things flowing chaotically about in our mind. When we open our eyes in the morning, our mind starts reorganizing all this, getting everything set up for the day. This puts us in a very vulnerable state, and we can easily spiral down a negative rabbit hole if we don't intentionally control our thinking, messing up the alpha and beta rhythm necessary to get us going, which, in turn, can make us depressed, anxious, and frustrated.

So, start each day self-regulating your thinking. This is what I do:

1. I capture any thoughts I'm thinking about as I wake up by using the 30–90 Second Rule.

2. I set my mind in the direction I want it to go. I focus on my mindset (for more on this, see my book *Think, Learn, Succeed*) and what I want to focus on during the day. These are some mindsets I have found useful in my own life, in my research, and in my clinical practice:

- I am determined to self-regulate my thinking, feeling, and choosing all day, which will help boost my intelligence, prevent cognitive decline, and reboot brain energy levels.

- I will not let any thoughts just wander chaotically through my mind today. I will be very analytical about capturing my thoughts.

- I will watch the words I say and recognize that they reflect my mind-in-action.

- I am the creator of my own emotions, so I can control my own emotions. I am not responsible for the cause of the emotion, but I am responsible for the expression of the emotion.

- I will stop being angry at the person who hurt me and work on forgiving them, because unforgiveness and bitterness can harm my brain and mental health.

- I will remember that happiness is not an end goal but part of the cycle of life. Often, happiness comes from embracing the tough, scary, and hard things life throws my way. It brings peace and it comes from deep inside my mind. Happiness is a choice.

- I will remind myself often that everything worthwhile takes time.

- I will always try to be open to multiple possibilities in any situation. Even when things don't go my way, I will be okay. Multiple attempts lead to multiple failures, which lead to multiple successes.

- I will choose to live in a state of gratitude and not focus just on what is going wrong in my life.
- I am designed for enhancement, not competition. When I feel the need to compete with someone or compare myself to others, I will remind myself that we need each other, and we need to celebrate our differences.
- I will make an effort to reach out and help someone today, because I know this will help me too. Supporting others, especially when I'm going through a tough time, can help clean up my own mental space.
- Today, I'll make my stress work for me and not against me. I know that the stress response will help me focus and think with clarity and flexibility.
- I will watch my expectations. Expectations influence my neurophysiology in a positive or negative direction.
- I know I have the ability to choose, which will change my brain structure right down to the genetic level. Today I will make choices that make sure this change goes in a healthy direction, because I control this process.

Try starting your day with mindsets like these for three weeks consecutively. This will help you start the day off well and help you tune in to your subconscious mind and get the alpha bridge working, which will connect to the theta and delta activity in the nonconscious mind. This, in turn, will help you pick up your emotional and physical warning signals (like anxiety, depression, heart palpitations, and mood swings) much quicker and mind-manage them. As we observed in our clinical trials, this kind of mind-management swing will help you feel more at peace during the day, giving you a feeling of contentment and autonomy.

2. Brain-Building Using the Neurocycle

As I mentioned earlier, brain-building is a great resilience-building, intelligence-boosting, mental mess–cleaning, and emotionally stabilizing exercise. It can be very spiritual and enriching, and can be done on a wide variety of content, from the news to spiritual study to knowledge needed to advance your education to anything you are interested in. Plan on spending fifteen to sixty minutes, minimum, spread throughout the day.

Using the 5 Steps for brain-building is a great way to boost your brain and mental health. I do this every day for at least one hour, and twice a day if possible. In fact, I use every opportunity I can to build my brain—it's a really good way to do some mental housekeeping and get rid of any toxic waste buildup, which affects my sleep and mental well-being.

Brain-building is also a great way to calm down, especially if you have just had a bad argument or are in a toxic situation. It restabilizes brain energy and chemicals, which often feel like they have been put in a blender when arguments and toxic things happen to us.

I normally do brain-building with my research, but I also do brain-building when prepping for podcast interviews, reading new books, watching educational videos, or catching up on the news. The process requires deliberate and intentional thinking, which gets us in that learning mode that's so vital to our mental and brain health. It really is like an energy boost—it makes you feel so good afterward. If I ever feel down, I'll do a quick brain-building session to get my theta and gamma rolling at increased amplitudes and my serotonin and anandamide (bliss hormones) flowing, which makes me feel so much happier and at peace.

Brain-building is also a great way to have more interesting discussions with people, especially those talks with people who have different viewpoints, which challenge you to get out of your comfort zone and really build up your mental bandwidth and resiliency.

3. Trauma and Habit Detoxes using the Neurocycle

I do my daily detoxes by neurocycling every day when I'm getting ready in the morning (showering, doing my hair, and putting on my makeup). This works for me because I like to detox before I dive into the day.

Detoxing through use of the 5 Steps, which takes seven to fifteen minutes a day, is a lifestyle. I'm always fixing something in my mind. We will never arrive at the perfect mental state. We should never become complacent or rest on our laurels, because life is all about growth. We should always be striving to improve our minds, and detoxing plays a large role in this because toxic thoughts are like a virus—they will penetrate everything and take over our mental space. You can also use my app to help you with this.

4. Thinker Moments

I do thinker moments throughout the day, for around five seconds to a couple of minutes every hour, when I'm tired, or for ten minutes around midday, in the sun if possible. I don't go a day without them because I don't do well without them. When we give our brain a rest by letting our mind wander and daydream, we reboot our brain and give ourselves that edge we need, helping us get in touch with that deeper, nonconscious, almost spiritual part of us.

Thinker moments are super easy to do, but in today's busy world we have to train ourselves to do them. All you have to do is close your eyes, sit back (or lie down), and relax. Just a few seconds will do the trick, but that ten- to fifteen-minute block in the sun is the best. You can also add a meditation routine to your thinker moments if you want, or take a couple minutes three to five times during the day to play and laugh.

5. Active Reaches

Active Reaches, done seven times throughout the day for one to three minutes each, are quick and easy to do and are the application part of the Neurocycle. They can be as easy as reading an Active Reach statement you've set as a reminder for yourself. This action keeps whatever you're reconceptualizing into a new thought in the conscious mind and gives it a good dose of energy every day, which helps it keep changing and growing stronger.

Remember, without these daily doses, your new, healthy thought won't become a habit and won't change your behavior. This process takes sixty-three days at least.

6. Eat Real Food Mindfully

As I mentioned in the last chapter, my only rule when it comes to eating is to eat real food mindfully. This means not only being aware of what we eat but also how we eat and why we eat. How we eat affects our thinking and, most importantly, how we think affects how we eat. Our internal environment is influenced by our mind, and this includes our digestive system. For example, your mind influences how effectively neuropeptides are released in the pancreas for the assimilation and digestion of food, so if you're in a toxic, messy mental state, this can affect the bioavailability of the nutrients and how well your digestive system functions overall, which can affect how you feel mentally and physically.

It doesn't matter what we eat as long as we strive to eat in a way that's mindful, with a diet that is made up of real, whole, and sustainable foods. There are plenty of great books, recipes, and meal plans out there that are centered around real, whole foods, so check them out.

7. Moving and Thermal Exercise

We all know the amazing benefits of exercise. I spend around forty-five to sixty minutes every day working out, and sixty to ninety minutes in my Sunlighten infrared sauna (or "thermal exercising," as they call it). I follow this with a cold shower.

Of course, as with food, there's no one way to exercise, and we all have unique needs and capabilities. The one thing that's important is that you get your mind into the game when it comes to exercise. As with eating, we need to exercise mindfully to get its full benefits. In fact, it's very hard to find an exercise routine and stick to it without doing some serious mind work.

I also like to incorporate movement into my day as much as possible. I always try to run up all the stairs we have in our house and do little workouts in between work, especially when I feel that brain fog moving in, like a quick power walk, some planks, or a few jumping jacks. When it comes to exercise, *all movement is good movement*!

8. My Sleep Routine

Sleep preparation begins in the morning when you open your eyes and continues all day. In fact, the neurocycling sleep routines I mentioned in the previous chapter all help me sleep better because they help me manage my mind better.

And when I can't sleep, I don't worry about it. I use the time to do what I didn't get to during the day or read a book, and I relax my mind. Worrying about not sleeping is one of the worst things you can do. Your body will cope, and you'll get through the next day. We're always complaining about how there are not enough hours in the day, so look at the times you can't sleep as more hours you can use to do what you want to do.

○ ○ ○ ○

As you have seen throughout this book, the mind-management of thoughts is the key to cleaning up the mental mess. This has been the overriding message and objective of all my work and research. I'm more passionate about the power of the mind now than when I first started out!

How you use your mind to manage your mind is incredibly important. It's the foundation of a happy and healthy life because it helps you make the choices that lead to a happy and healthy life. It doesn't mean you won't be troubled or never experience pain, discomfort, anxiety, or sadness. However, it does mean you can feel and experience all life has to offer and all life throws your way. It means you have the power to withstand acute events, daily stressors, and toxic people, because you now have the ability to clean up your mental mess. Mind-management is, in my opinion, one of the most important tools—if not the most important—in your mental toolbox, because it will help you live a longer, healthier, and happier life.

So, go forth and neurocycle!

Thank you! I'm very excited for this! I am on day 19 of my first cycle, and this has been the best investment I've ever made in myself. I am starting to break a lifelong habit of fear and anxiety. I can't wait to see what changes will be coming.

JANE

Appendix A

The Geodesic Information Processing Theory

I have researched the mind-brain connection and the science of thought over thirty years, creating what I call The Geodesic Information Processing Theory (see image in color insert). This theory is based on the neurophysiology of the learning process and has been demonstrated to improve academic performance by a conservative measure of 35 to 75 percent.

Essentially, The Geodesic Information Processing Theory describes the science of thought, stating that there are three levels: (1) nonconscious metacognitive level; (2) conscious cognitive level; and (3) symbolic output level. The nonconscious metacognitive level, where 90 to 99 percent of the action in your mind is, operates at four hundred billion actions per second, twenty-four hours a day, and drives the conscious cognitive level. The conscious cognitive level, where up to 10 percent of the mind action is, operates at two thousand actions per second, and when we are awake it drives the symbolic output level. Finally, the symbolic output level incorporates the five senses with which you receive information from the outside world and by which you express yourself, through speech or writing for example. Thoughts cycle through the three levels from nonconscious metacognitive to conscious cognitive to symbolic output, and vice versa. As thoughts cycle through the three levels, they change—and change the thoughts connected to them in a dynamic interrelationship.

The Geodesic Information Processing Theory is explained more fully in my peer-reviewed journal article, "The Development of a Model for Geodesic Learning" (University of Pretoria, 1997). For more information, see my book *Think, Learn, Succeed*, chapter 22.

Appendix B

The Metacog

A Metacog is a way of writing that closely resembles a tree-like structure, hence a thought. It really gets the two sides of the brain working together, and therefore the nonconscious mind, by drawing on the detail to big picture and big picture to detail. Using a Metacog is a great way of getting emotional, informational, and physical information out of the nonconscious mind. Below are abbreviated instructions for creating one; I suggest you look at the image below as you read through them, which will make it easier.

- Be creative and spontaneous—it doesn't have to be a neat work of art, and everyone's Metacog will follow the same basic principles but will look different.
- Start by writing the name of the thought you are working on in the center of your journal page or blank piece of paper.
- Put the first subheading on a branch that radiates out of the central bubble. Now just start writing the memories associated with this subheading of the thought.

- Try to keep each word on its own line, and try to write only about 30 percent of a sentence down—don't write in full sentences. This will help you get to the root of the issue more quickly. So, for example, instead of writing "I feel sad because I had an argument with X," rather write "Sad? = argued with X."

- Where you can, keep one word per line/branch—look at the example below. You literally build a sentence on branched lines, one word per line. If this doesn't make sense, draw a bubble and write as many words as you need in the bubble.

- The information radiating from the subheadings progresses from general to more specific. This means that you "grow" branches outward from the subheading

- Write on the line, not next to the line or under the line or in a bubble next to the line

The shape of the branches you are growing on your Metacog is, in a sense, matching the branches you are growing in your brain on the dendrites. The dendritic arbor in your brain is being reflected as a branched Metacog on paper. Without your being consciously aware of it, your neural network will dictate the shape of the branches on your Metacog. That's why I like to say that a Metacog is your "brain on paper." It's as though, as you draw it, your brain has already created the same pattern as a memory.

Use colors, images, arrows—whatever—especially at the Recheck phase to help you reconceptualize.

Remember, you build a Metacog, which means you are building a memory into dendrites.

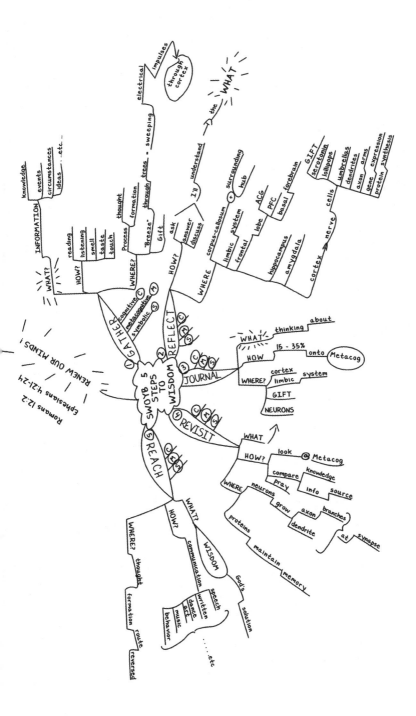

NOTES

Chapter 1 What Happens When We Don't Use Our Minds Correctly

1. Stephen M. Rappaport, "Genetic Factors Are Not the Major Causes of Chronic Diseases," *PLoS ONE* 11, no. 4 (April 2016): e0154387, https://doi.org /10.1371/journal.pone.0154387; World Health Organization, "Genes and Human Diseases," https://www.who.int/genomics/public/geneticdiseases/en/index2.html; Bruce H. Lipton, *The Biology of Belief: Unleashing the Power of Consciousness, Matter & Miracles* (Carlsbad, CA: Hay House, 2010); Deepak Chopra and Rudolph E. Tanzi, *The Healing Self: A Revolutionary New Plan to Supercharge Your Immunity and Stay Well for Life* (New York: Harmony, 2020).

2. Colin D. Mathers and Dejan Loncar, "Projections of Global Mortality and Burden of Disease from 2002 to 2030," *PloS Med* 3, no. 11 (November 2006): e442, https://doi.org/10.1371/journal.pmed.0030442.

3. Atul Guwande, "Why Americans Are Dying from Despair," *New Yorker*, March 23, 2020, https://www.newyorker.com/magazine/2020/03/23/why-americ ans-are-dying-from-despair; Olga Khazan, "Middle-Aged White Americans Are Dying of Despair," *Atlantic*, November 4, 2015, https://www.theatlantic.com /health/archive/2015/11/boomers-deaths-pnas/413971/?gclid=Cj0KCQjw6PD3B RDPARIsAN8pHuFA_qzt_odTW66Bat6l3cCLEX6w2v6j3TOnHS8−J7TsejFfR zxZRS4aAm5cEALw_wcB.

4. Colin D. Mathers and Dejan Loncar, "Updated Projections of Global Mortality and Burden of Disease, 2002–2030: Data Sources, Methods and Results," (Geneva: World Health Organization, 2005); Steven H. Woolf and Laudan Y. Aron, "The US Health Disadvantage Relative to Other High-Income Countries: Findings from a National Research Council/Institute of Medicine Report," *JAMA* 309, no. 8 (February 2013): 771–72, doi:10.1001/jama.2013.91.

5. Sibile Marcellus, "Certain American Men Are Dying 'Deaths of Despair,'" *Yahoo Finance*, October 22, 2019, https://finance.yahoo.com/news /deaths-of-despair-why-this-group-of-americans-has-higher-mortality-rates -130633528.html; Carol Graham and Sergio Pinto, "The Geography of Desperation in America: Labor Force Participation, Mobility Trends, Place, and Well-Being," Brookings, October 15, 2019, https://www.brookings.edu/research

/the-geography-of-desperation-in-america-labor-force-participation-mobility
-trends-place-and-well-being/?utm_campaign=Brookings%20Brief&utm_source
=hs_email&utm_medium=email&utm_content=78166038.

6. Graham and Pinto, "Geography of Desperation in America."

7. Woolf and Aron, "US Health Disadvantage."

8. Quishi Chen et al., "Prevention of Prescription Opioid Misuse and Projected Overdose Deaths in the United States," *JAMA Network Open* 2, no. 2 (2019): e187621–e187621.

9. Chen, "Prevention of Prescription Opioid Misuse."

10. Anne Case and Angus Deaton, "The Epidemic of Despair: Will America's Mortality Crisis Spread to the Rest of the World?" *Foreign Affairs* 99 (2020): 92; Anne Case and Angus Deaton, "Deaths of Despair Redux: a Response to Christopher Ruhm," Princeton, January 8, 2018, http://www.princeton.edu/~deaton/downloads/Case_and_Deaton_Comment_on_CJRuhm_Jan_2018.pdf.

11. Stephen Castle, "Shortchanged: Why British Life Expectancy Has Stalled," *New York Times*, August 30, 2019, https://www.nytimes.com/2019/08/30/world/europe/uk-life-expectancy.html.

12. Kristen L. Syme and Edward H. Hagen, "Mental Health Is Biological Health: Why Tackling 'Diseases of the Mind' Is an Imperative for Biological Anthropology in the 21st Century," *Yearbook of Physical Anthropology* 171, no. S70 (April 2020): 87–117, https://doi.org/10.1002/ajpa.23965.

13. Syme and Hagen, "Mental Health Is Biological Health."

14. Tom C. Russ et al., "Association between Psychological Distress and Mortality: Individual Participant Pooled Analysis of 10 Prospective Cohort Studies," *BMJ* 345 (2012): e4933; Alexander Michael Ponizovsky, Ziona Haklai, and Nehama Goldberger, "Association between Psychological Distress and Mortality: The Case of Israel," *J Epidemiol Community Health* 72, no. 8 (2018): 726–32.

15. Syme and Hagen, "Mental Health Is Biological Health."

16. United Nations, "Statement by Dainius Puras, Special Rapporteur on the Right of Everyone to the Enjoyment of the Highest Attainable Standard of Physical and Mental health," United Nations Office of the High Commissioner, October 29, 2019, https://www.ohchr.org/EN/NewsEvents/Pages/DisplayNews.aspx?NewsID=25203&LangID=E.

17. Awais Aftab, "Psychiatry and the Human Condition: Joanna Moncrieff," *Psychiatric Times*, April 10, 2020, https://www.psychiatrictimes.com/qas/psychiatry-and-human-condition-joanna-moncrieff-md.

18. Aftab, "Psychiatry and the Human Condition."

Chapter 2   What Is Mind-Management and Why Do We Need It?

1. Molly C. Kalmoe et al., "Physician Suicide: A Call to Action," *Mo Med* 116, no. 3 (2019): 211–16, https://www.ncbi.nlm.nih.gov/pmc/articles/PMC6690303/.

2. "Keith Ward - The New Atheists (Part 1)," YouTube video, 37:32, posted by ObjectiveBob, August 29, 2012, https://www.youtube.com/watch?v=fkJshx-7l5w&t=3s.

3. To learn more about the Wim Hof method, visit https://www.wimhofmethod.com.

4. "Neurofeedback," *Psychology Today*, accessed August 21, 2020, https://www.psychologytoday.com/us/therapy-types/neurofeedback.

5. Marc R. Nuwer and Pedro Coutin-Churchman, "Topographic Mapping, Frequency Analysis, and Other Quantitative Techniques in Electroencephalography," in *Aminoff's Electrodiagnosis in Clinical Neurology*, 6th ed. (2012), 187–206, https://www.sciencedirect.com/topics/medicine-and-dentistry/quantitative-electroencephalography.

Chapter 3 Why the Neurocycle Is the Solution to Cleaning Up Your Mental Mess

1. "Suicide Facts," Suicide Awareness Voices of Education, accessed August 20, 2020, https://save.org/about-suicide/suicide-facts/.

2. Find more information and download my Neurocycle app at neurocycle.app.

3. Ryan McVay, "Think It Takes 21 Days to Make a Resolution a Habit? Triple That," *NBC News*, January 2, 2014, https://www.nbcnews.com/health/body-odd/think-it-takes-21–days-make-resolution-habit-triple-n2881.

4. Phillippa Lally et al., "How Are Habits Formed: Modelling Habit Formation in the Real World," *European Journal of Social Psychology* 40, no. 6 (2010): 998–1009.

5. Chun Siong Soon et al., "Unconscious Determinants of Free Decisions in the Human Brain," *Nature Neuroscience* 11, no. 5 (2008): 543–45; Stuart Hameroff and Roger Penrose, "Consciousness in the Universe: A Review of the Orch OR Theory," *Physics of Life Reviews* 1 (2014): 39–78; Stuart Hameroff et al., "Conduction Pathways in Microtubules, Biological Quantum Computation, and Consciousness," *Biosystems* 64, no.1 (2002): 149–68.

6. Elizabeth Blackburn and Elissa Epel, *The Telomere Effect: A Revolutionary Approach to Living Younger, Healthier, Longer* (New York: Hachette, 2017); Elissa Epel, "How 'Reversible' Is Telomeric Aging?" *Cancer Prevention Research* 5, no. 10 (2012): 1163–68; Nicola S. Schutte and John M. Malouff, "The Relationship between Perceived Stress and Telomere Length: A Meta-Analysis," *Stress and Health* 32, no. 4 (2016): 313–19; Elissa S. Epel et al., "Wandering Minds and Aging Cells," *Clinical Psychological Science* 1, no. 1 (2013): 75–83; Elissa S. Epel, "Psychological and Metabolic Stress: A Recipe for Accelerated Cellular Aging?" *Hormones* 8, no. 1 (2009): 7–22; Elissa S. Epel et al., "Cell Aging in Relation to Stress Arousal and Cardiovascular Disease Risk Factors," *Psychoneuroendocrinology* 31, no. 3 (2006): 277–87; Naomi M. Simon et al., "Telomere Shortening and Mood Disorders: Preliminary Support for a Chronic Stress Model of Accelerated Aging," *Biological Psychiatry* 60, no. 5 (2006): 432–35; Christine G. Parks et al., "Telomere Length, Current Perceived Stress, and Urinary Stress Hormones in Women," *Cancer Epidemiology and Prevention Biomarkers* 18, no. 2 (2009): 551–60.

Chapter 4 The Research

1. Caroline Leaf, "Cleaning Up Your Mental Mess: Clinical Pilot Study on the Impact of Mind-Management to Deal with Depression, Anxiety and Toxic Thoughts," under review, NYP; Caroline Leaf, "Psychometric Testing of a

Knowledge, Attitudes, and Skills Instrument Related to Individual Self-Regulation for Depression and Anxiety: The NeuroCycle Questionnaire," under review, NYP.

2. Johann Hari, *Lost Connections: Uncovering the Real Causes of Depression—and the Unexpected Solutions* (London: Bloomsbury, 2019); Alaina J. Brown et al., "Feeling Powerless: Locus of Control as a Potential Target for Supportive Care Interventions to Increase Quality of Life and Decrease Anxiety in Ovarian Cancer Patients," *Gynecologic Oncology* 138, no. 2 (2015): 388–93; S. L. Slabaugh, M. Shah, and M. Zack, "Leveraging Health-Related Quality of Life in Population Health Management: The Case for Healthy Days," *Popul Health Manag* 20, no. 1 (2017): 13–22; Michael H. Antoni et al., "How Stress Management Improves Quality of Life after Treatment for Breast Cancer," *Journal of Consulting and Clinical Psychology* 74, no. 6 (2006): 1143; Johann Hari, "Is Everything You Think You Know about Depression Wrong?" *Guardian*, January 7, 2018, https://www.theguardian.com/society/2018/jan/07/is-everything-you-think-you-know-about-depression-wrong-johann-hari-lost-connections.

Chapter 5 How Can All This Science Help You?

1. Mohd Razali Salleh, "Life Event, Stress and Illness," *The Malaysian Journal of Medical Sciences* 15, no. 4 (2008): 9; Pratibha P. Kane, "Stress Causing Psychosomatic Illness among Nurses," *Indian Journal of Occupational and Environmental Medicine* 13, no. 1 (2009): 28; Philip W. Gold, "The Organization of the Stress System and Its Dysregulation in Depressive Illness," *Molecular Psychiatry* 20, no. 1 (2015): 32–47; Ronald Glaser et al., "Stress-Induced Immunomodulation: Implications for Infectious Diseases?" *JAMA* 281, no. 24 (1999): 2268–70; Viviana Cavalca et al., "Oxidative Stress and Homocysteine in Coronary Artery Disease," *Clinical Chemistry* 47, no. 5 (2001): 887–92; Ahmed Tawakol et al., "Relation between Resting Amygdalar Activity and Cardiovascular Events: A Longitudinal and Cohort Study," *Lancet* 389, no. 10071 (2017): 834–45; Ahmed Tawakol et al., "Stress-Associated Neurobiological Pathway Linking Socioeconomic Disparities to Cardiovascular Disease," *Journal of the American College of Cardiology* 73, no. 25 (2019): 3243–55.

2. Abiola Keller et al., "Does the Perception That Stress Affects Health Matter? The Association with Health and Mortality," *Health Psychology* 31, no. 5 (2012): 677; Jeremy P. Jamieson, Matthew K. Nock, and Wendy Berry Mendes, "Mind over Matter: Reappraising Arousal Improves Cardiovascular and Cognitive Responses to Stress," *Journal of Experimental Psychology: General* 141, no. 3 (2012): 417.

3. Eva Bianconi et al., "An Estimation of the Number of Cells in the Human Body," *Annals of Human Biology* 40, no. 6 (2013): 463–71; Ron Sender, Shai Fuchs, and Ron Milo, "Revised Estimates for the Number of Human and Bacteria Cells in the Body," *PLoS Biology* 14, no. 8 (2016): e1002533.

4. Leaf, "Cleaning Up Your Mental Mess: Clinical Pilot Study."

Chapter 6 What Is the Mind?

1. Stuart Hameroff and Roger Penrose, "Consciousness in the Universe: A Review of the Orch OR Theory," *Physics of Life Reviews* 1 (2014): 39–78; Stuart Hameroff et al., "Conduction Pathways in Microtubules, Biological Quantum

Computation, and Consciousness," *Biosystems* 64, no. 1 (2002): 149–68; Stuart Hameroff, "Consciousness, Microtubules, and 'Orch OR': A Space-Time Odyssey," *Journal of Consciousness Studies* 21, nos. 3–4 (2014): 126–53; Stuart Hameroff, "How Quantum Brain Biology Can Rescue Conscious Free Will," *Frontiers in Integrative Neuroscience* 6 (2012); Stuart R. Hameroff, Alfred W. Kaszniak, and Alwyn Scott, eds., *Towards a Science of Consciousness II: The Second Tucson Discussions and Debates* (Cambridge: MIT Press, 1998); Hameroff and Penrose, "Consciousness in the Universe."

2. Hameroff and Penrose, "Consciousness in the Universe."

3. Hameroff et al., "Conduction Pathways in Microtubules."

4. Stuart Hameroff, "Quantum Computation in Brain Microtubules? The Penrose-Hameroff 'Orch OR' Model of Consciousness," *Philosophical Transactions of the Royal Society of London. Series A: Mathematical, Physical and Engineering Sciences* 356, no. 1743 (1998): 1869–96; Laura K. McKemmish et al., "Penrose-Hameroff Orchestrated Objective-Reduction Proposal for Human Consciousness Is Not Biologically Feasible," *Physical Review* E80, no. 2 (2009): 021912.

5. Eva Bianconi et al., "An Estimation of the Number of Cells in the Human Body," *Annals of Human Biology* 40, no. 6 (2013): 463–71, https://www.tandfonline.com/doi/abs/10.3109/03014460.2013.807878; https://www.smithsonianmag.com/smart-news/there-are-372-trillion-cells-in-your-body-4941473/.

6. Leaf, "Cleaning Up Your Mental Mess: Clinical Pilot Study."

7. Elissa S. Epel, "Wandering Minds and Aging Cells," *Clinical Psychological Science* 1, no. 1 (2013): 75–83; Elissa S. Epel, "Psychological and Metabolic Stress: A Recipe for Accelerated Cellular Aging?" *Hormones* 8, no. 1 (2009): 7–22; Naomi M. Simon et al., "Telomere Shortening and Mood Disorders: Preliminary Support for a Chronic Stress Model of Accelerated Aging," *Biological Psychiatry* 60, no. 5 (2006): 432–35; Elissa S. Epel et al., "Accelerated Telomere Shortening in Response to Life Stress," *Proceedings of the National Academy of Sciences* 101, no. 49 (2004): 17312–15.

8. Ibid.

Chapter 7 The Interconnected Mind

1. Benjamin Libet, "Do We Have Free Will?" *Journal of Consciousness Studies* 6, nos. 8–9 (1999): 47–57; Benjamin Libet, *Mind Time: The Temporal Factor in Consciousness* (Cambridge: Harvard University Press, 2004).

2. Chun Siong Soon et al., "Unconscious Determinants of Free Decisions in the Human Brain," *Nature Neuroscience* 11, no. 5 (2008): 543–45; Benjamin Libet et al., "Time of Conscious Intention to Act in Relation to Onset of Cerebral Activity (Readiness-Potential)," in *Neurophysiology of Consciousness* (Boston: Birkhäuser, 1993), 249–68; Patrick Haggard, "Human Volition: Towards a Neuroscience of Will," *Nature Reviews Neuroscience* 9, no. 12 (2008): 934–46.

3. "Kintsugi," Wikipedia, accessed August 20, 2020, https://en.wikipedia.org/wiki/Kintsugi.

4. Caroline Leaf, "The Mind Mapping Approach: A Model and Framework for Geodesic Learning," unpublished DPhil dissertation (Pretoria, South Africa: University of Pretoria, 1997).

Chapter 8 The 5 Steps of the Neurocycle

1. Susan Biali Haas, "Journaling about Trauma and Stress Can Heal Your Body," *Psychology Today*, December 7, 2019, https://www.psychologytoday .com/us/blog/prescriptions-life/201912/journaling-about-trauma-and-stress-can -heal-your-body.

Chapter 9 Directing Your Brain for Change

1. Jill Bolte Taylor, *My Stroke of Insight: A Brain Scientist's Personal Journey* (New York: Penguin Random House, 2009); Jill Bolte Taylor, "My Stroke of Insight," TED Talk, February 2008, https://www.ted.com/talks/jill_bolte_taylor _my_stroke_of_insight/up-next; James J. Gross and Lisa Feldman Barrett, "Emotion Generation and Emotion Regulation: One or Two Depends on Your Point of View," *Emotion Review* 3, no. 1 (2011): 8–16; Barbara L. Fredrickson, "What Good Are Positive Emotions?" *Review of General Psychology* 2, no. 3 (1998): 300–19.

2. Barbara Fredrickson, *Positivity: Top-Notch Research Reveals the 3-to-1 Ratio That Will Change Your Life* (New York: Harmony, 2009); Michael A. Cohn et al., "Happiness Unpacked: Positive Emotions Increase Life Satisfaction by Building Resilience," *Emotion* 9, no. 3 (2009): 361; Barbara Fredrickson et al., "Open Hearts Build Lives: Positive Emotions, Induced through Loving-Kindness Meditation, Build Consequential Personal Resources," *Journal of Personality and Social Psychology* 95, no. 5 (2008): 1045.

3. Fredrickson, *Positivity*.

4. Benjamin Libet, "The Timing of Mental Events: Libet's Experimental Findings and Their Implications," *Consciousness and Cognition* 11, no. 2 (June 2002): 291–99.

5. Florin Dolcos et al., "The Impact of Focused Attention on Subsequent Emotional Recollection: A Functional MRI Investigation," *Neuropsychologia* 138 (February 17, 2020), https://doi.org/10.1016/j.neuropsychologia.2020.107338.

6. "The Science behind the Wim Hof Method," accessed August 20, 2020, https://www.wimhofmethod.com/science.

Chapter 10 Why It Takes Sixty-Three Days of Neurocycling to Form a Habit

1. Deepak Chopra and Rudolph E. Tanzi, *Super Genes* (New York: Random House, 2015); Deepak Chopra and Rudolph E. Tanzi, *The Healing Self: A Revolutionary New Plan to Supercharge Your Immunity and Stay Well for Life* (New York: Harmony, 2020).

2. Mark R. Rosenzweig, Edward L. Bennett, and Marian Cleeves Diamond, "Brain Changes in Response to Experience," *Scientific American* 226, no. 2 (1972): 22–29; A. M. Clare Kelly and Hugh Garavan, "Human Functional Neuroimaging of Brain Changes Associated with Practice," *Cerebral Cortex* 15, no. 8 (2004): 1089–102; M. C. Diamond, "The Significance of Enrichment," in *Enriching Heredity* (New York: Free Press, 1988); M. C. Diamond, "The Brain . . . Use it or Lose It," *Mindshift Connection* 1, no. 1 (1996): 1; Marion Diamond and Janet Hopson, *Magic Trees of the Mind: How to Nurture Your Child's Intelligence,*

Creativity, and Healthy Emotions from Birth through Adolescence (New York: Penguin, 1999); Qiang Zhou, Koichi J. Homma, and Mu-ming Poo, "Shrinkage of Dendritic Spines Associated with Long-term Depression of Hippocampal Synapses," *Neuron* 44, no 5 (2004): 749–57.

3. Rodolfo R. Llinás, "Intrinsic Electrical Properties of Mammalian Neurons and CNS Function: A Historical Perspective," *Frontiers in Cellular Neuroscience* 8 (2014): 320.

4. Mark E. J. Sheffield and Daniel A. Dombeck, "Calcium Transient Prevalence across the Dendritic Arbour Predicts Place Field Properties," *Nature* 517, no. 7533 (2015): 200–04; Panayiota Poirazi and Bartlett W. Mel, "Impact of Active Dendrites and Structural Plasticity on the Memory Capacity of Neural Tissue," *Neuron* 29, no. 3 (2001): 779–96; Maya Frankfurt and Victoria Luine, "The Evolving Role of Dendritic Spines and Memory: Interaction(s) with Estradiol," *Hormones and Behavior* 74 (2015): 28–36; Phillippa Lally et al., "How Are Habits Formed: Modelling Habit Formation in the Real World," *European Journal of Social Psychology* 40, no. 6 (2010): 998–1009; David T. Neal et al., "The Pull of the Past: When Do Habits Persist Despite Conflict with Motives?" *Personality and Social Psychology Bulletin* 37, no. 11 (2011): 1428–37; Benjamin Gardner, "A Review and Analysis of the Use of 'Habit' in Understanding, Predicting and Influencing Health-Related Behaviour," *Health Psychology Review* 9, no. 3 (2015): 277–95; David T. Neal, Wendy Wood, and Aimee Drolet, "How Do People Adhere to Goals When Willpower Is Low? The Profits (and Pitfalls) of Strong Habits," *Journal of Personality and Social Psychology* 104, no. 6 (2013): 959.

Chapter 12 Neurocycling to Detox Trauma

1. Indrajeet Patil et al., "Neuroanatomical Correlates of Forgiving Unintentional Harms," *Scientific Reports* 7, no. 1 (2017): 1–10.

Chapter 13 Neurocycling to Break Bad Habits and Build Good Lifestyle Habits

1. As quoted in Hooseo B. Park, *The Eight Answers for Happiness* (Bloomington, IN: Xlibris, 2014).

2. Glenn Hutchinson, "Mental Health 101: How to Improve Your Mental Health without Going to Therapy," Glenn Hutchinson, Ph.D., accessed August 21, 2020, http://glennhutchinson.net/How-To-Improve-Your-Mental-Health.html.

3. Michael J. Poulin et al., "Giving to Others and the Association between Stress and Mortality," *American Journal of Public Health* 103, no. 9 (2013): 1649–55, https://pubmed.ncbi.nlm.nih.gov/23327269/.

4. Brett Q. Ford et al., "Culture Shapes whether the Pursuit of Happiness Predicts Higher or Lower Well-Being," *Journal of Experimental Psychology: General* 144, no. 6 (2015): 1053, https://www.apa.org/pubs/journals/features/xge-0000108.pdf.

5. Frank J. Infurna and Suniya S. Luther, "Resilience to Major Life Stressors Is Not as Common as Thought," *Perspectives on Psychological Science* 11, no. 2 (2016): 175–94.

6. Cell Press, "Gene Linked to Needing Less Sleep Identified," *ScienceDaily*, August 28, 2019, https://www.sciencedaily.com/releases/2019/08/190828111247.htm; Karen Weintraub, "Why Do Some People Need Less Sleep? It's in Their DNA," *Scientific American*, October 16, 2019, https://www.scientificamerican.com/article/why-do-some-people-need-less-sleep-its-in-their-dna/.

7. Michael Pollan, *In Defense of Food: An Eater's Manifesto* (New York: Penguin, 2008), 1–27.

8. Michael Pollan, *The Omnivore's Dilemma: A Natural History of Four Meals* (New York: Penguin, 2006), 84.

9. Elissa S. Epel, "Psychological and Metabolic Stress: A Recipe for Accelerated Cellular Aging?" *Hormones* 8, no. 1 (2009): 7–22; "Brain-to-Gut Connections Traced," University of Pittsburgh, *ScienceDaily*, May 18, 2020, www.sciencedaily.com/releases/2020/05/200518154939.htm.

10. John J. Ratey, *Spark: The Revolutionary New Science of Exercise and the Brain* (New York: Little, Brown, 2008); Kelly McGonigal, *The Joy of Movement: How Exercise Helps Us Find Happiness, Hope, Connection, and Courage* (New York: Penguin, 2019).

11. Christiane D. Wrann et al., "Exercise Induces Hippocampal BDNF through a PGC-1α/FNDC5 Pathway," *Cell Metabolism* 18, no. 5 (November 2013): 649–59, https://doi.org/10.1016/j.cmet.2013.09.008.

12. Kirk I. Erickson et al., "Exercise Training Increases Size of Hippocampus and Improves Memory," *Proceedings of the National Academy of Sciences* 108, no. 7 (2011).

13. Tina Ronn et al., "A Six Months Exercise Intervention Influences the Genome-Wide DNA Methylation Pattern in Human Adipose Tissue," *PLoS Genetics* 9, no. 6 (2013): doi:1371/journal.pgen.1003572.

14. Thais Russomano, "Gravity: Learning about Life on Earth by Going into Space—An Interview with Joan Vernikos," *Aviation in Focus-Journal of Aeronautical Sciences* 4, no. 2 (2013): 509; Carl W. Cotman and Berchtold C. Nicole, "Exercise: A Behavioral Intervention to Enhance Brain Health and Plasticity," *Trends in Neurosciences* 25, no. 6 (2002): 295–301.

15. McGonigal, *Joy of Movement*.

ABOUT THE AUTHOR

Dr. Caroline Leaf is a communication pathologist and neuroscientist whose passion is to help people see the power of the mind to change the brain, control chaotic thinking, and find mental peace. She is the author of *Switch On Your Brain*, *Think and Eat Yourself Smart*, *The Perfect You*, and *Think, Learn, Succeed*, among many other books and journal articles, and her videos, top-rated podcast, *Cleaning Up the Mental Mess*, and TV episodes have reached millions globally. She currently does extensive research and teaches at various academic, medical, corporate, and neuroscience conferences, as well as in religious institutions around the world. Dr. Leaf and her husband, Mac, have four children and live in Dallas.

Live a **Happier**, **Healthier** Life

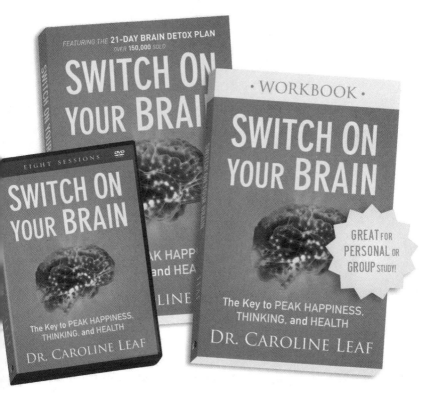

The bestselling book that has taught thousands how to achieve and maintain optimal levels of intelligence, mental health, peace, and happiness!

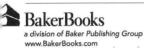

Tired of FAD DIETS, EMOTIONAL EATING, or POOR HEALTH?

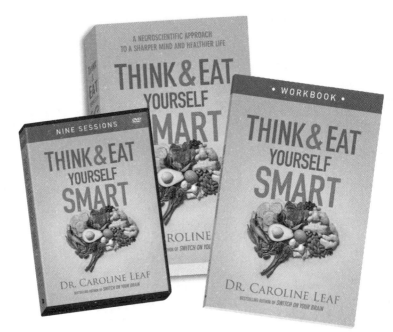

In this revolutionary book, Dr. Caroline Leaf packs an incredible amount of information that will change your eating and thinking habits for the better. Rather than getting caught up in fads, Leaf reveals that every individual has unique nutritional needs and there's no one perfect solution. Rather, she shows how to change the way you think about food and put yourself on the path toward health.

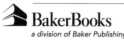

There is only
ONE YOU!

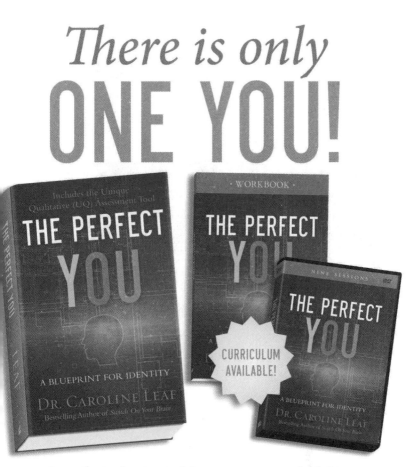

What is the **Perfect You?** It's how you process and exhibit your uniqueness through the way you think, feel, and choose. Everything you do and experience has an impact on the world, which is why it is vital for you to understand

- what your Perfect You is
- when you are stepping out of your Perfect You
- the mental, physical, and spiritual implications of stepping out of your Perfect You
- how to stay in your Perfect You

In this book, Dr. Caroline Leaf tackles this concept from theological, philosophical, and scientific angles, challenging you to think deeply about your identity and enabling you to apply these insights to your daily life.

UNLOCK YOUR
HIDDEN POTENTIAL

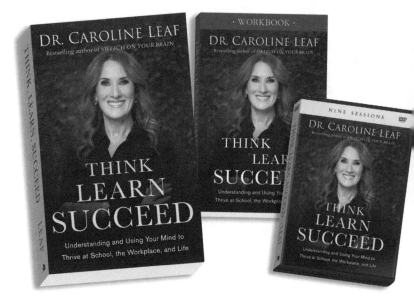

Backed by up-to-date scientific research and biblical insight, Dr. Caroline Leaf empowers readers to take control of their thoughts in order to take control of their lives. In this practical book, readers will learn to use

- The 5-Step Switch On Your Brain Learning Process, to build memory and learn effectively
- The Gift Profile, to discover the unique way they process information
- The Mindfulness Guide, to optimize their thought life and find their inner resilience

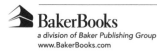

A HAPPIER, HEALTHIER, MORE ENJOYABLE LIFE—
STARTING TODAY!

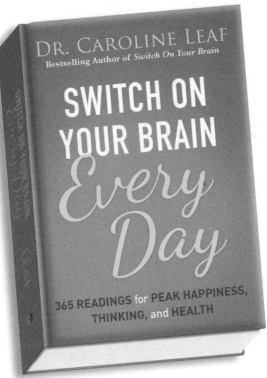

In her bestselling book *Switch On Your Brain*, Dr. Caroline Leaf offered a prescription for better health and wholeness through correct thinking patterns. Now she shows you how to instill the practices for living a healthy, happy life into your daily routine. These readings offer encouragement and strategies to reap the benefits of a detoxed thought life—every day!

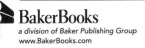

A Simple "How-To" Guide for
Improved Mental Health

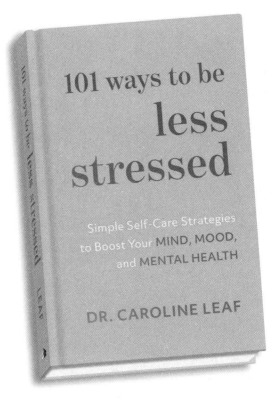

101 ways to be
less
stressed

Simple Self-Care Strategies
to Boost Your MIND, MOOD,
and MENTAL HEALTH

DR. CAROLINE LEAF

In this practical book, bestselling author and neuroscientist
Dr. Caroline Leaf reveals 101 simple and scientific ways to reduce
stress in order to boost your mind, mood, and mental health.
With these straightforward strategies for mental self-care, you
can change the way you think—and change your life.

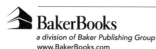

BakerBooks
a division of Baker Publishing Group
www.BakerBooks.com

Available wherever books and ebooks are sold.

Connect with
CAROLINE

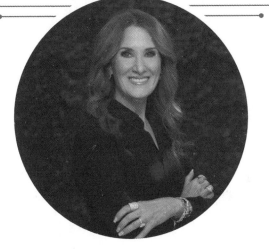

VISIT
DrLeaf.com

to learn more about Dr. Leaf and her
research, read her blog, listen to her podcast,
and follow her speaking schedule!

Also follow her on social media.

 drleaf

 DrCarolineLeaf

 drcarolineleaf

 Dr. Caroline Leaf

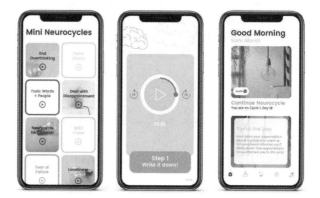
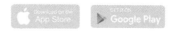

A TOP MENTAL HEALTH PODCAST
AROUND THE WORLD

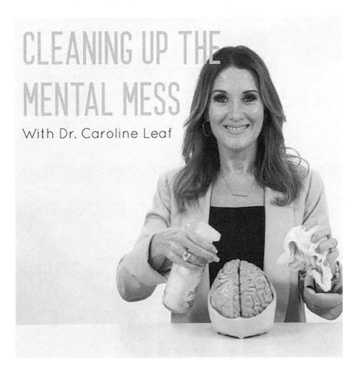

Tune in for practical tips and tools to help you take back control over your mental, emotional, and physical health.

Listen on Spotify, iTunes, PodBean, Anchor, YouTube, or DrLeaf.com.

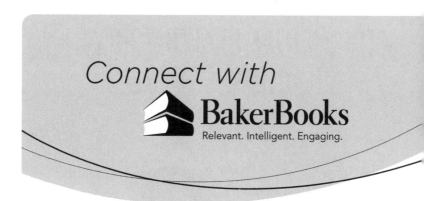

Connect with
BakerBooks
Relevant. Intelligent. Engaging.

Sign up for announcements about
new and upcoming titles at

BakerBooks.com/SignUp

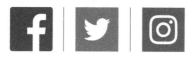

@ReadBakerBooks

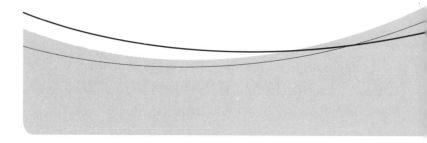